THE
TESTOSTERONE
FACTOR

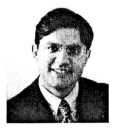

SHAFIQ QAADRI, MD, is a distinguished family physician, teacher, writer, and broadcaster. A gifted communicator, he has been a medical contributor to Canada's national newspaper *The Globe and Mail,* has published more than 700 articles on diverse health topics ranging from andropause to zinc deficiency, and has logged more than 500 radio and television appearances. Dr. Qaadri is one of the upper echelon Canadian MDs known as "Designated Medical Practitioners," and serves in the state legislature of the Government of Ontario. As a family physician for the past 15 years, Dr. Qaadri has advised, treated, and managed thousands of men going through andropause, and physicians and other healthcare professionals continually refer patients to his busy Toronto clinic. He is married with two children.

THE
TESTOSTERONE
FACTOR

SHAFIQ QAADRI, MD

THE
TESTOSTERONE
FACTOR

A PRACTICAL GUIDE TO
IMPROVING VITALITY AND
VIRILITY, *NATURALLY*

MARLOWE & COMPANY
NEW YORK

THE TESTOSTERONE FACTOR:
A Practical Guide to Improving Vitality and Virility, Naturally

Copyright © 2006 by Shafiq Qaadri, MD

Published by
Marlowe & Company
An Imprint of Avalon Publishing Group Incorporated

Library of Congress Cataloging-in-Publication Data

Qaadri, Shafiq.
The testosterone factor : a practical guide to improving vitality and
virility, naturally / Shafiq Qaadri.
p. cm.
Includes bibliographical references.
ISBN 1-56924-378-6
1. Testosterone—Therapeutic use. 2. Testosterone—Physiological
effect. I. Title.
RM296.5.T47Q33 2006
615'.366—dc22
2005030045

ISBN-13: 978-1-56924-378-7

Designed by Pauline Neuwirth, Neuwirth & Associates, Inc.

Printed in the United States of America

Contents

INTRODUCTION A Letter from the Doctor · xiii

PART 1 The Physical

1 BACKGROUND QUESTIONS · 3
2 SLEEP · 8
3 SEX · 18
4 EXERCISE · 33

PART 2 Internal Medicine

5 BACKGROUND QUESTIONS · 49
6 DIET · 55
7 HEART TROUBLE · 81
8 OBESITY · 95
9 DIABETES · 105
10 SUPPLEMENTS · 119
11 GENITAL AND URINARY SYSTEMS · 136

PART 3 External World—Your Mind and Outlook

12 BACKGROUND QUESTIONS · 151
13 STRESS LEVELS · 155
14 THERAPEUTIC SELF-MASSAGE · 171
15 WORKPLACE · 183
16 RELATIONSHIPS · 197
17 SPIRITUALITY AND HEALTH · 217
18 FINAL WORDS · 226

APPENDIX A: Full T-Questionnaire   229
APPENDIX B: Full T-Questionnaire Scoring Sheet   263
APPENDIX C: Full T-Questionnaire Scoring Explanation   264

Bibliography   277
Index   283

A Letter
from the Doctor

To the baby-boomer men who want to get more out of life,
Who want to be more vital,
And to those who love them . . .

I**T'S AN HONOR** to have this chance to speak with you directly. I'm also pleased to talk to you in plain language, so I don't have to hide behind my doc-talk, all those medical terms we've been taught to use, which often confuse people even more.

This is important, because the usual messaging from health practitioners doesn't seem to be getting through. Caregivers and their clients should all have such open and plain communication with each other more often.

First, baby-boomer men should be saluted. You boomers are the first generation to want it all—energy, vitality, creativity, grace under pressure, sensuality, good health, and well-being. You want to age vigorously and without disease. You want to be in your prime of life for as long as possible.

Women, Partners:

HELP YOUR MEN. After forty, our difficulties start. We men may become more irritable, and have our first heart attacks. We don't seek health care, and even if we do, we play down our concerns, don't ask questions, and can't remember the advice anyway.

We don't like to do tests. We just want to be told everything's fine. We won't take our supplements without reminders. We'll only get concerned about our health if we're in severe pain, or if we're

---

bleeding, or something's about to fall off—and sometimes not even then.

In fact, seven out of ten readers of health books, even the books about men's health, are women. We men, bless us, will only read about our own issues if our *significant other* recommends, threatens, or pleads with us to do so.

It's great that you are not content to see midlife as a time to start slowing down or fading away, letting the stresses of the world overpower you, accumulating problems like high blood pressure, diabetes, heart attacks, obesity, sexual problems, creaky bones, and weakening muscles. I heartily salute your desire for perpetual wellness. By doing so, you are waking up the medical establishment, and causing the world to take notice. You are forcing health practitioners to change their mind-set, to think in new ways, and to be promoters of health, not merely disease-catchers.

But here's the problem. What you may not realize is this—it's the effects of the master hormone that the body itself makes, testosterone (T), that can help put you at your best. Testosterone—made in the testes, controlled by the brain—promotes all the positive qualities, such as energy and vitality, just mentioned. In fact, testosterone has lifelong positive effects on your physique, emotions, intellect, relationships, behavior, and sexuality.

T is a true multitasking hormone.

But baby boomers are living longer than anyone in the history of humankind—men are now routinely living past the age of eighty. Men are pushing the limits, which is wonderful. I applaud all the developments that made it possible—in medical science, public sanitation, clean water, nutrition, antibiotics, immunization, and so on. Yours is the first generation to realize that aging does not have to be a slow decline.

But now I'll give it to you straight. If you're about forty-five years old or older—according to Nature—you're supposed to be dead already. That's what happened for generations up until the year 1900.

That's how it's always been for ages, and is still true today in many developing countries. It seems that we men were built for only a forty-five-year journey, not an eighty-year lifespan. We just aren't geared up for a service contract that runs so long—our lifetime warranty expires much earlier, but now our bodies have to work for an extra thirty-five years. The body's testosterone hormone production schedule, the communication routes, the distribution network, the whole arrangement we have going—it's all overextended.

It's like we're all hanging around after the party is over.

So we need to renegotiate our hormone service contract. Here's the story:

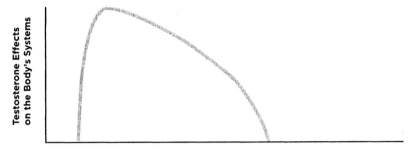

Graphically shown, the intensity of the Testosterone Effects on the Body's Systems follows this curve. First, there is an intense peak at puberty. Then there is a steady but accelerating decline, getting steeper with time, particularly at midlife.

On top of that, our modern lifestyle poisons the body: our nonrestful sleep, constant stress, never-ending demands on our time, attacks on our self-esteem, high blood pressure, excess weight, sitting around all the time, and dedicated eating of junk, cholesterol, sugar, and salt—all these damage our bodies.

The body's hormone-manufacturing ability is particularly hard hit. When your body is abused by the above factors, T is increasingly blocked from acting. It's neutralized, used up, burned off, wasted, or overwhelmed by competing, enemy hormones—which means you can't keep functioning at your best.

So what happens? Gradually, the body's hormone production systems run out of juice too early. And that's one of the core reasons for a wellness gap—why your *life span is longer than your health and well-being span.*

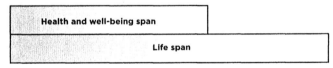

Graphically shown, your life span exceeds your health and well-being span

But it doesn't have to be this way. Hormones, the chemical messengers floating around in the blood, have always been there for you when it mattered.

Remember puberty, the transition to manhood, the coming of age, becoming a man—when hormones blew your mind? That was the doing of all the body systems working together, inspired and led by the brain–testes axis. It was a real power trip, one of the body's championship seasons.

Testosterone output was superspiked, giving you your beard, deeper voice, broader shoulders, bigger muscles, sexuality, new energy, ambitious personality, vigor, and a desire to take charge and take on the world.

GOOD TESTOSTERONE PRODUCTION is essential for adequate sperm production. At peak performance, we can make 3 million new sperm an hour.

Yet sperm counts in men today are *half* of what they were forty years ago. Men now account for the majority of infertility problems. This is another marker of the diminishing effects of testosterone.

After puberty, men more or less forget about the brain–testes axis. Indeed, most people don't have any idea of what this axis, this connected system, really does. The brain and testes talk to each other in a constant dialogue, monitoring each other's situation and needs. This axis, this workgroup, these partners, do much more for you than just sex and reproduction.

Men, you need to understand: to reach your full potential, you need to engage all the body's systems in a partnership, but you need to be especially aware of the much-neglected brain–testes connection.

Long after puberty, this axis can still do a tremendous amount, enhancing and upgrading your life. When the brain–testes connection is performing at *its* prime, so are you.

The testes can make billions of molecules of testosterone *per second*. It's like sending internal e-mails to every part of your body with instructions on what to do.

The brain commands and controls the testes. This hormone-manufacturing system, this internal chemistry production plant, can react with the speed of the stock market, in *real* time, based on what you are experiencing. Then when the brain gives the go-ahead, a magnificent flood of the T hormone is dispatched to act on every cell in every organ of the body—everywhere.

This hormone axis works on both your public and private parts. It's a whole department in operation that you aren't even consciously aware of while it is working behind the scenes for you, day to day, moment to moment.

The brain–testes department also wants to be in the business of building, solidifying, strengthening, and upgrading. But in this modern world, it seems all your testes' resources, all that precious T that is produced, gets used up just in repairing past damage. All the body's systems are simply running to keep in place. Little T is available for extras beyond basic maintenance, if that.

So it's time for some renewal, renovation, rescue, and servicing. Help your body's systems do what they were trained for, what they were born to do— which is to keep you energized, in your prime of life, with full vitality and virility.

Here's what you need to do:

- Refuse to just let yourself go and fade away.
- Respect your body's systems, and especially the brain–testes axis, with its testosterone (T) production capacity.

- Clear the way for T to work best.
- Commit to acting on this T-related information.
- Involve your partner as part of your team.
- Enjoy your newly enhanced vitality and virility.

One of your goals is to have your health and well-being span match your life span as much as possible:

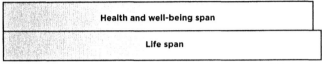

Graphically shown, ideally your life span matches your health and well-being span for as long as possible.

By following the protocols in this book, you will be able to change your testosterone-effects curve to look more like this:

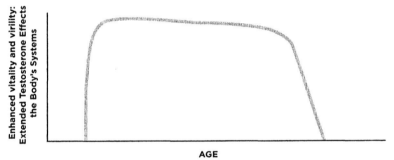

Graphically shown, ideally, the Testosterone Effects on the Body's Systems are extended, persistent, and prolonged. The intense peak at puberty is the same. But then there is a mostly steady state. Eventually, the curve does begin to decline, but this happens way beyond the midlife.

Thank you for this opportunity to be frank with you. I hope this book will help you to harness the power that is within you.

Yours in trust,

S. Qaadri, MD

THE
PHYSICAL

1

Background Questions

QUESTIONNAIRES ARE SCATTERED throughout this book. These self-tests give you a snapshot of how you're doing in a variety of areas—everything from Your Changing Body to Stress Levels to Your Changing Personality. These snapshots will help you to determine your particular areas of concern, and what recommendations you should especially follow.

ANSWERING QUESTIONS

Answer the questions honestly and in private. Answer in a way that's valid for you, and don't be influenced by anyone else's expectations. As a sample question, consider:

1. I wish I had taken better care of my health over the years.

❏	❏	❏	❏
0	*1*	*2*	*3*
None	*Mild*	*Moderate*	*Severe*

If you feel that this statement does not apply to you at all, check None.

Otherwise, if you feel this statement is valid for you, figure out how intensely you think it applies to you—Mild, Moderate, or Severe.

Depending on what you check—None, Mild, Moderate, or Severe—you are given a score—0, 1, 2, or 3 points.

BUILDING YOUR PERSONAL PROFILE

The questionnaires are usually tied to particular chapters that tell you how to deal with the difficulties discussed in their respective questions. However, as you work your way through the book, answering more questions, keep track of your point scores for each questionnaire; for instance, in the first three sections, you may score Mild, Moderate, or Severe. You will then begin to see an emerging profile of yourself.

Begin the physical assessment with this section, which contains the Your Changing Body questionnaire. This kicks off the background snapshot of your physical self. For now, think of your score rating—Mild, Moderate, or Severe—as how urgently you need to follow the recommendations in part 1. (If you want to know the full story right away, see appendices A, B, and C. But I recommend that you work your way through the book in the chapter order given.)

Then continue with the remaining chapters in part 1: Sleep, Sex, and Exercise.

—— Your Changing Body ——
(19 questions)

1. Are you becoming overweight, adding a new layer of fat around your waist?

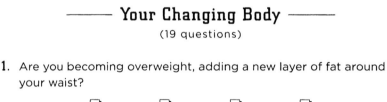

0	1	2	3
None	Mild	Moderate	Severe

2. Are you becoming overweight, developing a double chin?

0	1	2	3
None	Mild	Moderate	Severe

3. Are you catching colds, coughs, and infections more easily?

0	1	2	3
None	Mild	Moderate	Severe

4. Are you developing more allergies—new or worsening asthma, sinus problems, sneezing, or itchy rashes?

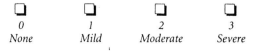

0	1	2	3
None	Mild	Moderate	Severe

5. Are you getting more and more skin wrinkles, dry skin, or sagging skin?

☐ | ☐ | ☐ | ☐
0 | *1* | *2* | *3*
None | *Mild* | *Moderate* | *Severe*

6. Are flesh wounds healing more slowly? ·

☐ | ☐ | ☐ | ☐
0 | *1* | *2* | *3*
None | *Mild* | *Moderate* | *Severe*

7. Are you rapidly graying or losing your hair?

☐ | ☐ | ☐ | ☐
0 | *1* | *2* | *3*
None | *Mild* | *Moderate* | *Severe*

8. Is the hair on your legs and chest thinning?

☐ | ☐ | ☐ | ☐
0 | *1* | *2* | *3*
None | *Mild* | *Moderate* | *Severe*

9. Do you feel you're experiencing more indigestion—more acid, heartburn, bloating, gas?

☐ | ☐ | ☐ | ☐
0 | *1* | *2* | *3*
None | *Mild* | *Moderate* | *Severe*

10. Are your gums becoming swollen and red, bleeding easily when you brush your teeth?

☐ | ☐ | ☐ | ☐
0 | *1* | *2* | *3*
None | *Mild* | *Moderate* | *Severe*

11. Are your breasts getting bigger, becoming more prominent—almost feminine?

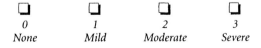

☐ | ☐ | ☐ | ☐
0 | *1* | *2* | *3*
None | *Mild* | *Moderate* | *Severe*

12. Are your legs and feet getting colder, leading you to wear socks more, even at night?

❑	❑	❑	❑
0	*1*	*2*	*3*
None	*Mild*	*Moderate*	*Severe*

13. Are you experiencing more joint stiffness?

❑	❑	❑	❑
0	*1*	*2*	*3*
None	*Mild*	*Moderate*	*Severe*

14. Are your muscles less flexible and more easily strained?

❑	❑	❑	❑
0	*1*	*2*	*3*
None	*Mild*	*Moderate*	*Severe*

15. Are you developing bad posture, slouching, hunching over, and not standing up straight?

❑	❑	❑	❑
0	*1*	*2*	*3*
None	*Mild*	*Moderate*	*Severe*

16. Do you feel like your bones ache deep inside?

❑	❑	❑	❑
0	*1*	*2*	*3*
None	*Mild*	*Moderate*	*Severe*

17. *Is this you?* "I've often got an aching neck, shoulders, or lower back."

❑	❑	❑	❑
0	*1*	*2*	*3*
None	*Mild*	*Moderate*	*Severe*

18. Do you feel your muscle strength is decreasing?

❑	❑	❑	❑
0	*1*	*2*	*3*
None	*Mild*	*Moderate*	*Severe*

19. *Is this you?* "I often ache all over, even though I didn't do that much activity. It's like my body's just been walloped."

❑	❑	❑	❑
0	*1*	*2*	*3*
None	*Mild*	*Moderate*	*Severe*

Your Changing Body

Your score:_____/ 57 points

Score/Rating:
0 to 6   *None*
7 to 23   *Mild*
24 to 46   *Moderate*
47 to 57   *Severe*

Consider your score range—is it None, Mild, Moderate, or Severe? Your score will help you determine how urgently you should follow the recommendations in the remaining chapters of part 1.

2

Sleep

I**T'S A QUESTION** we doctors ask all men. "So, how's your sleep?"
"Fine, thanks," they usually reply without much thought.
"Really?" we wonder.

—— Your Sleep ——
(9 questions)

1. *Is this you?* "I feel like I could always use more sleep."

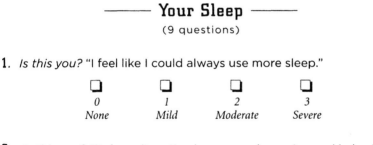

☐	☐	☐	☐
0	*1*	*2*	*3*
None	*Mild*	*Moderate*	*Severe*

2. *Is this you?* "It doesn't matter how many hours I spend in bed, I'm still not 100 percent the next morning."

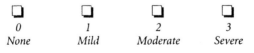

☐	☐	☐	☐
0	*1*	*2*	*3*
None	*Mild*	*Moderate*	*Severe*

3. *Does this happen often?* "I put my head on the pillow, and I toss and turn, waiting and waiting to fall asleep."

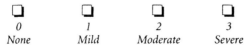

☐	☐	☐	☐
0	*1*	*2*	*3*
None	*Mild*	*Moderate*	*Severe*

4. *Is this you?* "When I get into bed to sleep, it's hard for me to turn off my thoughts. I've got too much going through my mind."

❑	❑	❑	❑
0	*1*	*2*	*3*
None	*Mild*	*Moderate*	*Severe*

5. *Is this you?* "The slightest little noise or movement wakes me up."

❑	❑	❑	❑
0	*1*	*2*	*3*
None	*Mild*	*Moderate*	*Severe*

6. *Is this you?* "I think I get less than six hours of *real* sleep every night."

❑	❑	❑	❑
0	*1*	*2*	*3*
None	*Mild*	*Moderate*	*Severe*

7. Do you wake up often in the middle of the night?

❑	❑	❑	❑
0	*1*	*2*	*3*
None	*Mild*	*Moderate*	*Severe*

8. *Is this you?* "I don't usually remember my dreams."

❑	❑	❑	❑
0	*1*	*2*	*3*
None	*Mild*	*Moderate*	*Severe*

9. *Is this you?* "For me to feel rested, I have to oversleep. I sleep in on the weekends, and get my catch-up rest."

❑	❑	❑	❑
0	*1*	*2*	*3*
None	*Mild*	*Moderate*	*Severe*

Your Sleep

Your score:_____/ 27 points

Score/Rating:

0 to 3   *None*

4 to 11   *Mild*

12 to 22 *Moderate*

23 to 27 *Severe*

Consider your score range here—is it None, Mild, Moderate, or Severe? Your score will help you determine how much you might benefit from this chapter.

THE IMPORTANCE OF SLEEP

SLEEP IS NOT about lying down, closing your eyes, and going brain-dead for a few hours. It's far more dynamic, full of internal activity. This includes a night-long hormonal distribution. The fact is, sleep is T-time. Men get their maximum testosterone exposure during sleep. Having too few hours of sleep, or having sleep that is not restful, robs them of their T-quota.

We live in a supercaffeinated, drive-through, pushbutton, always-open, touch-screen, leave-a-message, call-waiting, kiss 'n' fly, next-appointment, five hundred–channel world that is toxic to restful sleep. Armed with double lattes, it is no wonder that we suffer from a chronic sleep deficit.

Following these recommendations will help you get better sleep, thus maximizing your T.

Key Points
- Sleep promotes testosterone.
- At night, testosterone promotes sleep.

Sleep Differences Between Men and Women

IN NORTH AMERICA, women sleep on average 1½ hours more than men: 7½ hours for women, 6 hours for men.

This difference has a deep effect on quality of life, and the difference in life span—the longevity gap—between women and men.

SLEEP AND TESTOSTERONE

Testosterone is highest during sleep, and highest during the best part of sleep, known as REM sleep. The hormone starts rising when you go to bed, and peaks in the early morning at about dawn. (That's probably the time we should be getting up, biologically speaking, but we don't any longer, because of our modern lifestyle.)

That's why dawn is the most *fertile* time for a man, the best time to impregnate. You will spill the most sperm, and the best long-distance swimmers, at dawn.

These all-night hormone spikes are also why men will get multiple erections, lasting on average for fifteen minutes, the precise length of a testosterone release cycle. *Sorry, gentlemen, this happens when you're asleep.*

That's why men (should) wake up with erections.

SLEEP AND AGING

Men over forty have lighter and less restorative sleep. This results in declining T-levels.

Conversely, if aging men boost their T-production through the various means described in this book, one of the benefits will be a more restful and deeper sleep. This will snowball into even more T-production.

SLEEP, EMOTIONS, AND THOUGHTS

During sleep, you de-stress, rejuvenate your drive, and recharge your energy. It's when you refortify your ambition and creativity. It's when you fix yourself up and settle new ideas in the mind. These processes are all T-related.

WHAT TO DO

ALL MEN WILL benefit from any and all of the following steps. But those who had Severe scores in the Sleep questionnaire—23 to 27—should pay particular attention to these recommendations.

- Try to perfect your sleep.
- Follow the basics.
- Eliminate noise pollution.
- Eliminate light pollution.
- Ensure that your mattress and pillow are optimal.
- Sleep with the lower half of your body naked.
- Cool the room slightly.
- Get deep REM sleep.

TRY TO PERFECT YOUR SLEEP

Sleep is when you strengthen your bones, muscles, memories, blood, sperm, and new learning. It's when your onboard diagnostics and your immune system self-heal and detoxify. It's when you repair both physical and psychological wounds. It's when you grow both physically and psychologically.

Testosterone leads, triggers, oils, oversees, contributes to, mediates, or is involved in all of these restorative processes. The better you sleep, the more testosterone shines. As this hormone level rises, it also promotes other brain chemicals important for quality sleep—including, melatonin, serotonin, and human growth hormone.

Here is where the effect kicks in: the more refreshing your sleep, the more your body will not only produce more T and experience its benefits to greater effect, but also it will build a better production capacity for testosterone.

By the time you are forty-five years old, you will have spent one-third of your life asleep. That's about fifteen years—*years*—asleep. Make that time work for you.

Generally, men who follow these steps report that they spend less time in bed, and they don't waste so much time actually falling asleep, as they "sleep smarter," more efficiently, making better use of their time.

FOLLOW THE BASICS

For at least two to three hours before you sleep:

- No caffeine
- No large meals
- No strenuous exercise (sex is okay, though)
- No alcohol
- No nicotine
- No liquids

Caffeine, strenuous exercise, and nicotine are all stimulating, and wake people up. A large meal diverts blood and attention to the gut—away from, for example, the brain and testes. Alcohol may make you drowsy, but will interfere with the quality of sleep. It actually disrupts the pattern of high-quality sleep, known as the sleep architecture.

Also, drinking lots of liquids two to three hours before going to sleep almost guarantees that you will have to get up at night to urinate.

Still Getting Up to Urinate?

IF YOU FOLLOW these basic steps but still get up each night to urinate two or more times, it may be a sign of other problems—possibly diabetes or prostate enlargement.

If this is the case, talk to your health-care practitioner.

ELIMINATE NOISE POLLUTION

Wear Earplugs

There is a difference between quiet and silence. Sleep in *complete* silence.

You may think your bedroom is relatively noise free, but to optimize sleep, go the extra distance and get earplugs.

Take care to use proper earplugs, usually made of a light rubbery material that bends and molds to the shape of your ear canals. These are available from most pharmacies. Don't stick some homemade junk into your ear.

While wearing earplugs, you may not hear your alarm clock because your sleep is so deep. Make sure you have an alarm clock that is loud enough to hear through earplugs. Same for your smoke and carbon monoxide detectors.

All Quiet on the Western Front:

T EFFECTS ARE stronger in *complete* silence.

Your body thinks you are safe, interpreting silence as a stress-free zone.

ELIMINATE LIGHT POLLUTION

Electricity and lighting are relatively recent inventions. For centuries, men went to bed at sunset and rose at dawn. Now, we can have bright lights on at any hour of the day. Our bodies need continuously to adjust to this, playing havoc with our body's natural rhythms. No longer tied to the cycles of sunlight, our bodies suffer from light poisoning. That's great for night productivity but bad for quality sleep.

"But, doc, my room's totally dark," you may say. That may be true at night, but most homes will allow sunlight, moonlight, street light, and light from adjacent rooms to creep into the bedroom. We've seen all kinds of drapes, shades, blinds, and window covers, but none are completely impenetrable. Unless you have special hotel-quality window curtains called blackout covers, your room will have too much light. Even if you have these covers, perhaps during the night someone else in your home will turn the light on and defeat the purpose of the curtains.

Wear a Sleep Mask

There is a difference between dark and pitch-black dark. Sleep in *complete* darkness, by wearing an opaque sleep mask over your eyes to block out all light. These are also available from most pharmacies.

How Do I Look?

MEN APPRECIATE THE high quality of sleep they get from these two recommendations, earplugs and a sleep mask. But they have to put up with taunts from their spouses:

"Hey, you look like that guy Felix Unger, from *The Odd Couple*."

"Gee, how romantic. You look like you're inspecting nuclear waste . . . are you radioactive?"

"C'mon, you are not going to wear all that, are you? You look like you've been taken hostage."

We recommend that you soldier on, and remind your partner how she will benefit from *your* enhanced testosterone.

With *complete* silence and in *complete* darkness, you are undergoing a controlled sensory deprivation. This leads to a kind of lockout. Your body, mind, and brain will be able to completely disengage, shut out the constant self-chatter, distractions, thoughts, and background noises. This will encourage an absolute sleep.

ENSURE THAT YOUR MATTRESS AND PILLOW ARE OPTIMAL

Waking up sore, fatigued, and unrefreshed is a sign of decreased hormone impact throughout the night. Sleeping soundly on quality bedding induces testosterone production, which helps repair and maintain your body. Don't sabotage your T-levels by spending a third of your life on soft, cheap, or old bedding.

Some of my clients have had poor or interrupted sleep for years because of chronic back pain. Some thought that only back surgery would help. Yet they avoided any operation and obtained substantial relief just by changing to a firm, supportive mattress. After the switch, they didn't wake up achy, stiff, and unrested, which is what happened when they lay on inferior materials. They were amazed at how much better they slept after they spent a little more on a comfortable mattress and pillow.

Invest in a Good, Firm, Supportive Mattress and Pillow

The hotel industry understands this, and prides itself on its bedding. They invest large sums of money in firm yet compliant mattresses, which may even have special cushioned padding called pillow-tops.

You do *not* need to have a rocket-propelled mattress that vibrates, heats up, or moves to special positions—just buy a trusted brand that will keep its shape for a number of years.

TO MAINTAIN A good, flat sleeping surface, did you know that you should flip your mattress over every month or so? This eliminates compression, the downward curve in the cushioning that is caused by your body.

Make sure Your Bed Is Large Enough

If you are frequently disturbed by an acrobatic bed partner, get a bigger bed. Maybe you need a king-size? You might also wish to explore split surfaces (two twin beds joined by a king-size headboard) or special mattresses that don't allow one bed partner's movements on one half to disturb the other.)

Pets and children should sleep elsewhere, too.

SLEEP WITH THE LOWER HALF OF YOUR BODY NAKED

Wear a long shirt, a sports jersey, or an oversized T-shirt.

Give the testes what you've deprived them of all day—freedom. Then they will be able to set their own desired temperature without interference.

Got Kids?

SLEEPING IN THE nude from the waist down may not be practical if kids are around.

Lock the bedroom door. Keep a robe nearby.

Or be creative and figure out a solution that works for your situation.

COOL THE ROOM SLIGHTLY

Set your room temperature between 65 and 70 degrees Fahrenheit, and resist using heavy blankets and duvets. If you wake up feeling overheated and sweaty, or find you kick your covers off during the night, your room or covering is too warm.

Let the room be as cool as will allow you to sleep comfortably. Get a reliable digital thermometer that allows you to measure your bedroom temperature exactly—no more fiddling and guessing on rotary dials. (We like the fact that many new homes come equipped with digital thermostats, which give exact readings; even so, you should measure the temperature in your bedroom, not what may be happening in some other room where your heating system's thermostat may be located.)

> **Temperature Wars**
>
> OFTEN YOU AND your mate may not agree on the right bedroom temperature. Try to negotiate the coolest temperature that's suitable for both of you. Here is where separate tastes in blankets and other coverings may be an easy solution.

Why Sleep in a Cool Room?

Let's say the temperature is too hot, for example, 80 degrees Fahrenheit. Your body will sweat all night to try to cool off. That means that more warm blood is brought to the skin surface, presenting the body's internal heat to the outside. In this situation, there is a diversion of blood from the hot, inner core to the periphery. You're diverting that blood *away* from the testes, and thus reducing their ability to function to capacity. Not what you want.

Now let's say the temperature is too cool, down to 50 degrees Fahrenheit. In this scenario, your body's systems think, "It's way too cold in here. To heck with the unimportant bits, the skin, fingers, hands, feet, toes, earlobes, and whatever . . . I'm going to divert blood internally, to the most vital parts— brain, heart, and other organs, including the kidneys and testes."

This is what you want. By cooling the room, you can focus the blood flow to your vital organs, including the testes, making use of the body's natural ability to control and to redeploy blood flow to its various parts and systems. (This is the body skill that saves lives by shutting down blood flow to a cut limb, or keeping blood pressure up in times of severe bleeding.)

Obviously, it is unrealistic to expect you to have a good night's sleep in a 50 degree bedroom. However, you can achieve this reallocation of resources by sleeping at a comfortably cool temperature, between 65 to 70 degrees.

Stay cool.

GET DEEP REM SLEEP

Sleep from six to eight hours nightly.

This is the range of how much sleep that you actually need, not just the amount of time you spend in bed.

Deep REM Sleep is Testosterone-Sleep

Sleep experts talk about the five stages of sleep, the "sleep architecture." Basically, while you sleep you go through ninety-minute cycles, and the last fifteen minutes of each cycle are the restoring portions, provided you are sleeping deeply enough to have entered REM sleep. REM means rapid eye movement sleep. This is when you dream, as if your eyes were rapidly watching internally projected movies. We all dream every night during REM sleep, whether we remember the dream content or not.

It is during REM sleep—dream sleep—that we get a handle on our waking anxiety and challenges. This is when we imagine, when we play out possibilities, and when we can even solve perplexing problems creatively.

REM sleep is also the part of the cycle in which T peaks. This is when men have, on average, erections lasting fifteen minutes each, recurring throughout the night in each ninety-minute cycle.

The quality and amount of your REM sleep will affect every aspect of your physical and emotional state—including your sperm count, bone strength, ambition, drive, stress tolerance, irritability, and energy.

To maximize your REM sleep, follow the first seven sleep recommendations steps as best you can.

Avoid Sleeping Pills

PRESCRIPTION AND OVER-the-counter sedatives just knock you out. They actually decrease the amount of deep sleep, your REM T-time. Follow the seven suggestions, and you should achieve a satisfying sleep without the need for artificial aids.

HOW WILL YOU KNOW IF YOU'VE HAD GOOD-QUALITY SLEEP?

- When you put your head on the pillow, you didn't have to wait too long to go to sleep.
- When you went to bed, distracting thoughts turned off fast.
- Slight noises or movements did not stir you, disturb you, or wake you up.
- You did not wake up in the middle of the night. *Not even once.*

When you wake up the next day,

- you remember your dream(s).
- you don't feel that you need more sleep.
- you say, "Wow, I only slept for six hours, but it feels like a lot more."
- you're surprised that the achiness and fatigue you may have had the day before are *completely gone.*
- you don't want shoot your alarm clock.
- you feel a bounce in your spirit and think, "Bring on the day. It's good to be alive—I'm feeling 100 percent."

3

Sex

SEX, ORGASM, TESTOSTERONE—improve any one of these, and the other two automatically improve also.

Continue your self-rating by taking the quiz below and seeing where you stand.

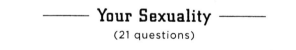

——— Your Sexuality ———
(21 questions)

Desire

1. Compared to when you were thirty-five, are you having sex less often?

❑	❑	❑	❑
0	*1*	*2*	*3*
None	*Mild*	*Moderate*	*Severe*

2. *Is this you?* "I'm having sex less often than I would *like*."

❑	❑	❑	❑
0	*1*	*2*	*3*
None	*Mild*	*Moderate*	*Severe*

3. Are you less horny, have less sexual desire?

❑	❑	❑	❑
0	*1*	*2*	*3*
None	*Mild*	*Moderate*	*Severe*

4. Do you feel less sexually aroused by your regular partner?

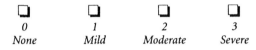

0	1	2	3
None	Mild	Moderate	Severe

Fertility

5. Are you having trouble conceiving either your first or second child because of sperm problems?

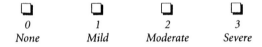

0	1	2	3
None	Mild	Moderate	Severe

Erections

6. *Is this you?* "When I used to wake up in the morning, I'd always have an erection. Now, not so much."

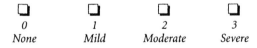

0	1	2	3
None	Mild	Moderate	Severe

7. *Is this you?* "I am *less confident* of getting an erection when I need one, and I worry about my sexual performance."

0	1	2	3
None	Mild	Moderate	Severe

8. Do you feel that your erections are weaker, less full-bodied, less sizable than they were?

0	1	2	3
None	Mild	Moderate	Severe

9. Do you frequently experience difficulty penetrating for sexual intercourse because of weak erections?

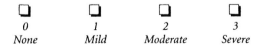

0	1	2	3
None	Mild	Moderate	Severe

10. *Is this you?* "During sex, I often lose my erection."

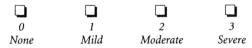

0	1	2	3
None	Mild	Moderate	Severe

11. Do you ejaculate (come) too soon?

| 0 | 1 | 2 | 3 |
| None | Mild | Moderate | Severe |

12. When you ejaculate, does less fluid come out?

| 0 | 1 | 2 | 3 |
| None | Mild | Moderate | Severe |

13. When you're having an orgasm, do you feel that the muscle contractions, the pulses, are weaker?

| 0 | 1 | 2 | 3 |
| None | Mild | Moderate | Severe |

Satisfaction

14. While you are having sex, are you worried that you might have a heart attack?

| 0 | 1 | 2 | 3 |
| None | Mild | Moderate | Severe |

15. Is your *partner* less sexually satisfied?

| 0 | 1 | 2 | 3 |
| None | Mild | Moderate | Severe |

16. Has the number or intensity of your *partner's* orgasms lessened?

| 0 | 1 | 2 | 3 |
| None | Mild | Moderate | Severe |

17. Has sex been less satisfying for *you*?

| 0 | 1 | 2 | 3 |
| None | Mild | Moderate | Severe |

18. *Is this you?* "I feel sexually *unsatisfied*."

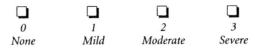

0	1	2	3
None	Mild	Moderate	Severe

19. Do you find that masturbating, self-pleasuring, is a more intense high than intercourse?

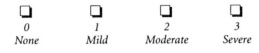

0	1	2	3
None	Mild	Moderate	Severe

20. *Is this you?* "Of course I have orgasms. But they're not as *powerful* anymore. I am not as sensitive down there. It's like I'm thinking, "Yeah, we had sex, but is that *it*?"

0	1	2	3
None	Mild	Moderate	Severe

21. *Is this you?* "Sexually, I was always ready to go, ready to rock. But now we've got to do all this stuff to get me up and going—I need a lot more stimulation. I really miss the old days. Where's the magic gone?"

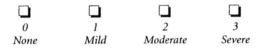

0	1	2	3
None	Mild	Moderate	Severe

Your Sexuality

Your score:_____/ 63 points

Score/Rating
0 to 6   None
7 to 25   Mild
26 to 50   Moderate
51 to 63   Severe

Consider your score range here—is it None, Mild, Moderate, or Severe? This score will help you determine how much you may benefit from the recommendations in this chapter. You will improve your sex life by practicing these suggestions, thus maximizing the benefits of T.

In fact, understand this—the testosterone concentration in the testes is one hundred times the concentration of testosterone in the blood. This is remarkable, unheard of in biological systems. It's as if the testes are a super-vault, a Fort Knox.

Sex is the force that accesses this storage vault, the blast that releases some of this T into the circulation. The testicles swell during sex by about 50 percent, and they're just waiting for the testosterone to be harvested.

Whatever else you think you may be doing during sex, that's the main biological benefit that the body is after.

Key Points

- Sex promotes testosterone.
- Testosterone promotes sex.
- Orgasm promotes testosterone.
- Testosterone promotes orgasm.

Sex as an Elixir

MEN WHO HAVE more sex, and more intense orgasms, live longer.
They even *smile* more.
These are both T-benefits.

Sex is a testosterone storm.

Sex is therapeutic.

Sex is one of the most special things that a man can do. It's powerful, a sign of energy, an expression of intimacy, a way to bond deeply, a way to lose yourself in someone else. It's a workout, and a heck of a T-rush.

Some men think of sex as a physical experience, others feel it's spiritual. Either way, the body loves the chemistry of sex.

For most men, it's also the most exercise they ever do.

THE CHEMISTRY OF SEX

ANTICIPATING SEX INCREASES testosterone, and having sex releases T into the bloodstream throughout the whole body. Sex juices you up, revving up the hormones, circulation, and electrical nerve firing.

During sex, more than six times the normal blood flow goes into the penis to make it erect. This is incredible. Nothing else in the body comes close.

Also, the testes swell with blood and fluid to about 1½ times their usual size.

Finally, testosterone explodes throughout the body during orgasm.

The Sweet Smell of Success:

MEN AND WOMEN give off their own musk, their own sexual scents known as pheromones. These scents are derivatives of testosterone in *both* men and women.

You are supposed to give off more pheromones as you build your T. The cosmetic industry is devoting huge resources to research and commercialize these scents.

That sex does all these things is the reason men can be so affected by sexually charged things—a beautiful person, sheer clothing, a toned physique, sleek hair, nudity, a memory-triggering perfume, a romantic song, a sultry voice, a youthful face, a seductive smile, or curves in the right places.

Good, energetic sex, or slow, leisurely loving—both help to release large amounts of T, which in turn releases endorphins, the body's own pleasure chemicals and onboard painkillers.

WHAT TO DO

- Get enough sex.
- Get better-quality sex, beyond just routine.
- Self-service when necessary.
- Learn to masturbate each other.
- Go oral.
- Learn the power of suggestion.
- Get kinky.
- Don't always be so goal oriented.
- Open up.
- Deal with any erection trouble.

GET ENOUGH SEX

How many times are you supposed to have sex to optimize your testosterone levels? Men are always asking this question, and there's no one answer that's right for everyone.

First, when I say to have sex, I mean to reach orgasm. Biochemically speaking, the body doesn't seem to mind if you have an orgasm with a partner or alone. Either way seems to give off a good T-rush.

"I'm All Hot and Bothered for Nothing."

IDLE FLIRTATIONS CAN be particularly annoying to a man's chemistry. It's like showing men the menu but not letting them eat.

Biochemically, during arousal, testosterone is building up locally within the testes, and the body is waiting for its release via orgasm, expecting a rush. But if it's not released as anticipated, it's as if the body goes into a mini-withdrawal, giving up the T-hit for that encounter.

Try to Have Sex at Least Every Five to Six Days

The sperm themselves are expecting to come out into the world at least every five to six days. Any less than that seems to send a signal to the brain that sex and testosterone building are not priorities. It's as if the brain thinks you're ungrateful for your sperm, because you're not sending them forth as fast as they're being made. The brain then slows down signaling, and this diminishes T production levels.

Sperm, for example, will die if they sit in the testes for more than six days. If a man doesn't ejaculate at least that often, there will be excess numbers of dead sperm coming out—the ones who missed an earlier outbound flight and died waiting for the connection.

Do It Almost Daily

This is a guideline based on what works for most clients.

Having given you the range, what I've found is this: Men who have an orgasm more or less daily do the best. So, if you're up for it, a once-daily discharge is recommended.

Don't Overdo It

On the other hand, try not to have an orgasm more than once per day. Regularly having sex more than once per day, for any sustained period of time, is extremely tiring. Usually men beyond their teens only keep up that kind of schedule during their honeymoon.

Learn to Have Quickies

Consider it sport sex.

No one has much time for anything these days, and that can include sex. You may be too tired, too busy, have an early day tomorrow, the kids aren't asleep yet, and so on.

If you can squeeze a quickie into your routine once in a while, not necessarily at bedtime, your body will appreciate it. For example, let's say you're both getting ready to go out to dinner. You may find yourselves alone, about to get dressed—there's your window.

Sex doesn't always have to be some grand production, with music, soft lighting, and a romantic prelude. Sometimes efficient sex is all you'll have time for, just a shared physical experience. Now, this shouldn't become your *routine*, because your partner won't appreciate it.

GET BETTER-QUALITY SEX, BEYOND JUST ROUTINE

Warm Up Beforehand

Do a five- to ten-minute warm-up before you're about to have sex. This is a remarkably simple thing, but powerful. It's just like the warm-ups you do before exercise. Walking on the spot, light jogging, floor stretches—all of these will enhance sex by getting your blood flowing and pumped with oxygen.

Cultivate Variety

Try different positions, locations, and lingerie. Anything to break the monotony. T doesn't spike as intensely when you have settled into a routine that no longer excites you.

There are any number of lovemaking manuals, whether it's the original *Kama Sutra*, the Indian book of lovemaking, or more updated guides and videos, or satellite television. Experiment with and find new positions and angles that allow deeper penetration, longer intercourse, and deeper pleasure.

Try different thrusts, become a bit of a teenager again. Don't always do what you always do. Do what you've always wanted to do. Try some seemingly impossible positions.

> SOME MEN USE this instruction as a justification for having an extramarital affair.
>
> Let me be clear. That may be what your body chemistry is prompting you to do, but that is *not* my recommendation.
>
> The idea is to rediscover excitement with the partner you already have.

Extend Foreplay

The longer you engage in foreplay, the more your testosterone percolates, boils, rises, and builds in anticipation. And then the release is more intense. There is no officially recommended duration, of course. That's an individual choice. But make a conscious effort to prolong your before-intercourse play. Don't make every act a quickie—you'll be depriving your partner, and also depriving your own body of a much-deserved supersize jolt of T.

Teach your partner to stimulate your testes during foreplay. Access some of that T that's brewing at one hundred times the concentration found in the blood.

Post-Fight Sex

Anger T + Sex T = a big rush.

You have probably heard, or know from your own experience, that you get a certain hormonal rush right after an argument. Testosterone released by anger can then mix and amplify the T released by sex.

In fact, post-fight sex can increase a man's T-release by anywhere from 10 to 45 percent. Again, the whole body then benefits.

So consider having sex right after an argument. You're going to have to work off that steam somehow. Try it sometime.

Couples actually surprise each other by the intensity of sex at this time. In fact, one of the biggest T-rushes is having sex when you're angry.

Note that this is *not* a recommendation to promote rage as a form of foreplay, to sexually abuse your partner while angry, or to insist upon sex if your partner is unwilling following a spat. *If* you have had an argument, *and it has ended*, a sexual reconciliation *may* be in order.

SELF-SERVICE WHEN NECESSARY

> I'm such a good lover because I practice a lot on my own.
> Don't knock masturbation, it's sex with someone I love.
> —*Woody Allen*

"I was shocked. My husband thought I was sleeping, but I wasn't. He was playing with himself . . . right there in our bed. I was . . . I don't know, hurt and angry. It was strange. Why does he need to do that if I'm around?"

It is estimated that 70 to 80 percent of married men masturbate with some regularity.

Now, if their partner asks, "You don't do this, do you?" they will likely say no. They'll reply, "No, not me." They will frown, as if to say, "How could you think such a thing? How could you accuse me of this?" But he is masturbating on occasion. Really. Partners, keep in mind that his masturbating is good for both of you. It sets off a T-release, which benefits those times you make love together.

"It's More Intense."

The expression of sexuality is part of being a full human being. And the desire continues even if your spouse is not available, or if you would rather just pleasure yourself once in a while.

Spouses have a hard time accepting this, but men do continue to masturbate even after marriage. Neither of you should be ashamed: it's merely biology percolating to the surface.

Men report that when they self-pleasure their orgasm is more intense than when they have intercourse. Biochemically, that means their T-rush is greater.

Why?

When masturbating, men control all the motions, pressure, rhythm, touch, warmth, and gyrations exactly according to what they like. It's a time of tremendous concentration toward one goal only.

LEARN TO MASTURBATE EACH OTHER

Note that the preceding recommendation is to be exercised *occasionally*. If you are in a relationship, as a couple you and your partner will both benefit by learning how to pleasure each other, how to take sex to new heights with new approaches. This will also remove some of the performance anxiety you may be experiencing.

Enlarge your sexual repertoire by learning how to manually stimulate each other.

GO ORAL

"I love her so much for trying to do this. I know she didn't want to at first."

Some spouses are shocked or appalled when we suggest this.

But some men have been looking for its justification: "See, even the doctor said this is what I need."

Men love receiving oral sex. Few have had as much or as skillful oral sex as they want, certainly not from the person they're married to.

Partners, think of it as one of the many options besides usual intercourse. Oral sex is one of them.

LEARN THE POWER OF SUGGESTION

Talk dirty to each other in unexpected places or times. Tell each other about the sex you'll have later in the day. Send each other naughty messages on a PDA or BlackBerry. T builds in anticipation.

Learn to blow each other's minds.

GET KINKY

This isn't for everyone, certainly. But some couples are usually ready to try some new additions to their lovemaking.

There is an endless variety of erotica—lubricants, massage oils, toys, music, and vibrators. Sometimes just heating your regular moisturizer cream and using that on your partner is enough. There are even creams available that heat up on skin contact.

Try watching a sensual film together—not alone.

> MEN WHO GIVE sperm samples for infertility testing are usually given some erotic material for inspiration, either a film or magazine. It has been demonstrated that they will release more sperm if they sex themselves up. This is the result of an enhanced T-spike, as their brain responds to the sexually stimulating material.

DON'T ALWAYS BE SO GOAL ORIENTED

Slow Down

Women complain that men are too quick to move to intercourse, to move to penetration. From a testosterone-release point of view, they're right.

The longer you extend foreplay and go through the preliminaries, the more aroused you will become. That leads to a higher build up of T, and consequently a more explosive release and distribution of T throughout the body upon orgasm.

Learn not to be so fast; don't always play the hungry lion waiting to go in for the kill. Good sex is not always about reaching orgasm quickly. You'll have more of a T-release if you just relax, letting things build naturally.

Savor Your Sexual Encounters

Stop time-pressuring each other, or making sure the other person is totally getting off. Just be with each other in a suspended time zone, letting the feelings flow, enjoying the many sensations of your bodies.

Also, men report that they don't always have to have an orgasm, they don't always have to ejaculate, to experience fulfilling sexual pleasure.

But we do recommend that men have an orgasm, as that's the major event that releases T throughout the body. More satisfying sex can increase a man's T-release by anywhere from 10 to 35 percent. Then the whole body benefits.

TEACH EACH OTHER

"I don't know what my girlfriend has been reading, but she's so much more into having sex. . . . Before, it only seemed like kind of a duty."

Both partners should use their whole bodies. Don't let one partner just be an observer or receiver. Share with each other what turns both of you on. Encourage your partner to return your caresses and explore the many sexual zones of your body; likewise, learn and respond to your partner's desires. Be open to suggestions. Do whatever you can to add to the sensory experience, rather than concentrating only upon the genital area.

Demonstrate How You Feel

For men, their *partner's reaction to their lovemaking* is just as much of a high for them as the sex itself.

So, partners—verbalize, moan, scream, whisper sweet nothings—whatever it takes to heighten your excitement and aid communication. Place a hand or guide lips to what you feel needs extra attention. Don't expect your partner to magically know whether to speed up or slow down; use sound and motion to say, "You're getting warmer."

Don't wait to be asked later if it was good. *Make* it good.

Also, outside the times you spend in actual sexual engagement, partners who maintain a trusting dialogue with each about what pleases them sexually have more fulfilling sex.

Understand that learning to give and receive better sex is a health matter, as well as a means to enhance your relationship.

During times other than your actual engagement in sexual activity, tell each other what works for you sexually. Be open, honest, and sensitive to the other person's needs. Everybody is turned on by different things, and responds differently. Try to word criticisms and requests in a positive way. If your partner is uncomfortable engaging in suggested activities, don't force the issue; learn more about and work with what does turn your partner on. Your overall relationship is more important than the pursuit of an activity you are really not enjoying together.

WHEN THERE'S ERECTION TROUBLE

"We were about to make love, but I noticed I wasn't hard enough. I was too embarrassed to say, 'Dear, would you mind getting me hard.' I let a few minutes go by, and obviously my wife was wondering why I wasn't going in and taking the plunge. I kept stroking her, hoping as she enjoyed herself, and kind of wriggled next to me, that I would get hard as I usually would have. But it wasn't happening.

"I started to think more about my erection than about her—get hard, get erect, stand at attention. I started to think about some other experiences, I imagined I was making love to [favorite actress], but nothing. I just stayed sort of erect, full of promise, but not good enough to penetrate.

"Then my wife turns to me, trying to be all consoling-like. 'It's all right,

Robbie, it can happen.' I was polite about it, but I was angry and humiliated. I just felt like a loser. 'Damn,' I thought, 'This doesn't happen to me.' That day I learned that all those commercials for Viagra and all that talk we keep hearing was real. Another one bites the dust."

The Importance of Communication

"Now we talk about our sex together . . . It's so refreshing to do this. He wants to pleasure me, and I want to do the same. What a difference a little dialogue makes. I have no idea why it took us so long to talk openly about such an important area of our lives."

When sexual difficulties arise, that's when having open channels of communication and honest talk help the most. You can share your anxieties, work on solutions together, and preserve your self-esteem.

Otherwise, men may start avoiding sex, hope that their erection problems will just go away, or ask for secret prescriptions of Viagra or its cousins.

Keeping the cross-talk open will let you feel unthreatened and not humiliated. This is the first step in helping to deal with performance anxiety.

Otherwise, anxiety and damaged self-esteem can kill future erections. You become so afraid it will happen again that it becomes a self-fulfilling prophecy.

Erection Problems Are Common

Your age determines the chance that you will have some form of erection problems. If you're fifty years old, for example, you have a 50 percent chance of having difficulties. We estimate that about 35 million men in North America have some degree of erection problems.

Beyond these statistics, it means that such difficulties are massively widespread. So, if you have been experiencing this, be assured that you are not alone.

> AS MEN AGE, especially if they have not catered to their T, they will lose sensitivity in their genitals. They will have slower electrical nerve firing, and diminished blood supply.
>
> It's important to know that, in this situation, the man needs more direct caressing of his genitals to result in a full erection.
>
> Anticipate that this will occur naturally with age, and learn what may work for you and your partner to strengthen and maintain your erections.

The Leading Causes of Erectile Dysfunction

The leading causes of erection problems are also the leading causes of diminished testosterone:

- High cholesterol
- High blood pressure
- Heart disease
- Diabetes
- Smoking
- Obesity
- Lack of exercise
- Chronic stress

Erectile Dysfunction (ED) May Be a Sign of Heart Trouble or Blockages Elsewhere

Most erection problems are caused by partially blocked arteries, the same kind of cholesterol and plaque blockages that cause heart attacks. In addition, doctors are now learning that erection problems are often a clue to circulatory blockages elsewhere than the heart.

The opposite is also true. There is increasing evidence that high cholesterol and heart blockages are often a precursor of erection problems.

Erection Pills

If a man needs to use Viagra or its cousins to achieve an erection, that's a practical solution that should not be treated as an embarrassment. Having a firmer erection for better sex will lead to a more intense testosterone storm during orgasm.

Following the T-building strategies in this book will also increase your sensitivity to these medications, making for a more intense orgasm and enhanced sexual desire. Definitely explore enhancing your sex life with the suggested strategies. Why?

It's an interesting fact that erection pills don't work without the engagement of the brain. You won't get an erection just by sitting there, even if you have taken a pill. Your brain must receive and respond to stimuli. These pills make you more responsive to sexual thoughts and stimuli.

This is just like what happens with testosterone—it's the brain that places the orders for T in response to sexual thoughts and stimuli. So don't depend on just a pill to get you going—becoming more involved in your overall sensations will boost your T and help the drug do its job.

WARNING: Erection pills are to be *absolutely avoided* if a man is using nitrates, usually prescribed for chest pain (angina) treatment. If you use both together, you can collapse from too low blood pressure.

Heart Disease and Erections

SEX, ERECTILE DYSFUNCTION (ED) medications, and T all release NO, nitrous oxide, a substance that dilates blood vessels and increases blood flow. Consequently, such drugs as Viagra, Levitra, and Cialis are being studied for their potential as heart pills.

WHAT GOES AROUND COMES AROUND

IN SUMMARY, A vigorous, warm, and rewarding sex life will build T-capacity and T-release.

The testosterone that bathes your body during sex will in turn help you with your sexual arousal, desire, pleasure, orgasm, responsiveness, and sensitivity.

That same T will have beneficial effects on your body's other systems. Sex doesn't only feel good, it's good for your health.

4

Exercise

HAVE HEARD a lot of excuses to get out of exercise.

One of the best was from a distinguished fifty-three-year-old gentleman. "Pelvic *what?* I can't do that, I'm a tax accountant."

What's Your Excuse?

"Who has the time to go off to some gym?"

"I'm too tired at the end of the day to exercise."

"I've got to get to work in the morning."

"I'm too out of shape."

"I'm too old for that nonsense."

The majority of men—some 60 percent—do no regular exercise at all. They only change the location of where they're sitting—from their home to their car to work to a meeting and then back home. This is especially true of men in midlife, when demands on their time can become overwhelming. Yet this is the group that can benefit from these exercises the most.

——— Your Appearance ———
(5 questions)

1. Are you less pleased with how you look?

    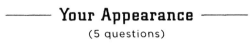

0	*1*	*2*	*3*
None	*Mild*	*Moderate*	*Severe*

2. Are you less concerned than you used to be with grooming, with your facial hair and hairstyle?

0	*1*	*2*	*3*
None	*Mild*	*Moderate*	*Severe*

3. *Is this you?* "I used to get more positive attention because of my physical appearance, and this bothers me."

    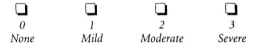

0	*1*	*2*	*3*
None	*Mild*	*Moderate*	*Severe*

4. Have you seriously thought about plastic surgery to enhance your self-image?

0	*1*	*2*	*3*
None	*Mild*	*Moderate*	*Severe*

5. Are you concerned that you're looking *too old too fast*, aging before your time?

0	*1*	*2*	*3*
None	*Mild*	*Moderate*	*Severe*

Your Appearance

Your score:_____/ 15 points

Score/Rating
0 to 2   *None*
3 to 6   *Mild*
7 to 12   *Moderate*
13 to 15   *Severe*

────── Your Energy Levels ──────
(5 questions)

1. Are you feeling lazier, with less get-up-and-go?

☐ ☐ ☐ ☐
0 1 2 3
None *Mild* *Moderate* *Severe*

2. Do you fatigue quickly?

☐ ☐ ☐ ☐
0 1 2 3
None *Mild* *Moderate* *Severe*

3. *Is this you?* "I fall asleep when I don't mean to—when I'm watching TV, or right after dinner."

☐ ☐ ☐ ☐
0 1 2 3
None *Mild* *Moderate* *Severe*

4. Do you *feel* older than your actual age?

☐ ☐ ☐ ☐
0 1 2 3
None *Mild* *Moderate* *Severe*

5. *Is this you?* "My stamina has really gone down over the last couple of years."

☐ ☐ ☐ ☐
0 1 2 3
None *Mild* *Moderate* *Severe*

Your Energy Levels

Your score:_____/ 15 points

Score/Rating
0 to 2 *None*
3 to 6 *Mild*
7 to 12 *Moderate*
13 to 15 *Severe*

Consider your score ranges here for the questionnaires Appearance and Energy Levels—did you score None, Mild, Moderate, or Severe? Your scores here help you determine how urgently you need the recommendations in this chapter.

In fact, by increasing circulation and helping to "clean the pipes," exercise enhances the pick up of testosterone from the internal production facilities, helping to deliver T to all the body's tissues, leading to a huge number of benefits, not only for your appearance and energy levels. This effect is particularly supported by exercise in *moderate* amounts *regularly*, using pelvic-focused exercises.

Follow the recommendations here, to benefit from this systemwide tune-up.

Key Points
- Exercise enhances the production, release, requirement, and distribution of testosterone.
- This effect on T is vastly superior if you exercise in *moderate* amounts *regularly* using pelvic-focused exercises.

WHAT TO DO

- Stop Making Excuses. Find time. Do Something.
- Do Pelvic Cardio Exercise.
- Do Pelvic Resistance Exercise.
- Learn What Your Body Says to Itself When You Exercise.
- Fidget.

STOP MAKING EXCUSES. FIND TIME. DO SOMETHING.

We have heard them all. Men waste a lot of time making up excuses not to exercise. The internal thinking goes like this: "Just wait till this project is done, or this quarter is over, or once the year-end results are in, or after I get through this busy time, or after I quit smoking, or when summer starts, or before the insurance physical, or during vacation, or right after New Year's . . ."

In this manner, most men rob themselves of the benefits of exercise. Stop making excuses.

Find Time
Three things that often stop men from exercising are:

1. They overplan. They take on too much, especially when pretending to plan to exercise. Men think they can accomplish more than

they do. They find they might have ten or fifteen minutes, not the originally estimated one or two hours. Rather than use their limited time constructively, nothing gets done.

2. They lose their initial enthusiasm to exercise. Men will sign up at the gym or purchase fancy equipment, exercise for the first few weeks, and then just stop. Men forget that owning equipment or signing up for a gym membership doesn't necessarily mean they will exercise.

3. Waiting for a special time to exercise. By not making exercise part of your rhythm, part of your normal routine, it does not get done.

Stop looking for excuses to neglect your body. Make exercise a habit. If you have to, actually schedule exercise into your calendar, just as you would with any other appointment.

Do Something

Some men admit up front that they're not the "exercising kind."

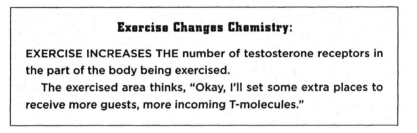

Exercise Changes Chemistry:

EXERCISE INCREASES THE number of testosterone receptors in the part of the body being exercised.

The exercised area thinks, "Okay, I'll set some extra places to receive more guests, more incoming T-molecules."

One fellow said, "I know I'm supposed to do all this. I've got a bunch of these exercise brochures and some DVDs. My wife keeps giving them to me. But I hate them . . . I can't imagine anything so boring."

Fine. If you can't follow a particular program, find physical activities that you do like, and make those your exercise. Choose ones that you enjoy, because if you don't like them, you won't do them. These may include dancing, gardening, playing friendly tennis or squash, climbing stairs, walking in the evening, walking on the golf course, brisk window-shopping at your favorite mall, extra-long or fast walks with your dog, playing with your children, or just walking in place as you watch television (you don't need a special step machine to do this).

For example, walk faster and more deliberately. Exaggerate your steps and straighten up, as if you're marching in the military or in a parade. When you stop at a light, contract the muscles of your hands, arms, buttocks, thighs, and calves. Walk with perfect upright posture.

Use ten or fifteen spare minutes. Just stand up wherever you are, anywhere, and start walking on the spot. Exercise even if you're tired. Whenever possible, choose to walk instead of driving or taking the bus.

We have seen that even small measures work well, *if done regularly.* You don't have to be a trained athlete who only works out at top-level gyms with personal trainers to get the benefits of exercise.

Be creative. Find yourself opportunities to be active. But begin at a pace that you can handle, and build up your exercise capacity step by step—don't try to walk five miles on the first effort. Trying to do too much too soon is one way you might become discouraged.

How Often Do You Need to Do Specific Exercises?

I recommend exercising between two and five times per week. Generally, more is better, as long as you don't overstrain yourself. If you score in the Severe range, you should definitely consider maximizing your exercise regimen, up to five times per week. But it is also key to do these exercises regularly. If it's just twice a week, but you exercise unfailingly, that will be better in the long run than waffling between spurts of activity and weeks spent on the sofa. Your developing muscles need to stay toned to work for you, and the lapse of more than a few days can undo all the progress you've made.

DO PELVIC CARDIO EXERCISE

Why does exercise that gets your heart pumping make you feel better?

Inside the testes, testosterone is made on the side roads, in the narrow pathways, in the wilderness, as it were. Sperm are made on the main roads, and get the prime location on main highways.

When you do a cardiac workout, you send more blood rushing through the testes. The extra waves of blood wash through to those side roads where testosterone is waiting to be rescued.

Remember: Within those side roads of the testes, testosterone is concentrated at one hundred times the usual blood levels. There's oil in them there hills. Pelvic cardio exercise pumps it out.

That's one of the reasons cardiac exercise, as opposed to other regimens, increases testosterone so fast—why you feel good quickly, and why that feeling lingers. A good heart workout helps T-collection and T-dispersal.

How Often Should You Do Pelvic Cardio Exercise?

Fifteen minutes is a minimum suggestion for a pelvic cardio program. Ideally, it's part of a larger cardiac workout. But even if it isn't, it can be enormously beneficial.

The Jumping Squat

The jumping squat is one of the best all-around exercises.

1. Stand up straight, legs apart.
2. Jump down to a squat. Hands are on the ground. Knees are touching your chest. You're crouching.
3. Throw your legs back as if you are about to do a push-up. Hands are still on the ground supporting you.
4. Bring knees forward again to the same crouch position as in step 2. Knees are touching your chest again. Hands are still on the ground supporting you.
5. Jump up, standing straight and tall again.

This is tough, and a real workout. It hits more than just the pelvic area.

How many do you have to do? Aim for a baseline of four sets of ten repetitions.

The Air Bicycle

1. Sit on a sturdy chair with armrests. Make sure you have good back support. Do not sit on a bicycle for this. Sitting on the ground works too, but a sturdy chair with armrests is better.
2. Start pedaling in the air. Vary the circles you make. Imagine that you're traveling on different terrains and at different speeds. Use small, quick pedaling circles for sprints; large, full arcing circles for going up hills.

Keep your legs further apart than you normally would, more than if you were on a real bike. Don't squish the scrotum, which is where you're sending the rushing blood to with this exercise.

You need a baseline of five minutes of air-bicycle exercise. This is tough. Take as many legitimate breaks as you need. But the total pedaling time should be a minimum of five minutes.

The Pelvic Thrust

"You mean air sex, doc?"

Yes.

1. While standing in a slight squat, hands on hips, act like a male stripper. Thrust your pelvis back and forth, in your best heave-ho, one-two, I'm-giving-it-to-you-now movement.

You can modify this:

> 2. Stand with one foot forward, one foot back, as if you're about to lunge like a fencing champion. Thrust back and forth as before.

This second position actually allows for much wider movement, and men find this more comfortable.

This exercise does look obscene, so some family members may be scandalized. Especially onlooking kids.

You need a baseline of three minutes for this exercise.

Pelvic Circles

"You trying to teach me how to belly dance?"

Yes. That's what it looks like.

> While standing, slightly squatting down, hands on hips, move your pelvis in wide, wide circles. Remember the hula hoop—same type of movement.

One client reported his wife's comment: "You look like you're in heat, waiting to jump the first thing that comes by."

Despite its amusing appearance, this exercise also gives some rotational movement for the spine, which is unusual for most exercise regimens. This helps with nerve conduction and balance sensors as well as with T production and delivery.

You need a baseline of three minutes for this exercise.

Suggested Pelvic Cardio Workout Schedule:

1. First set of jumping squats, 10 repetitions.
2. The air bicycle, 5 minutes.
3. Second set of jumping squats, 10 repetitions.
4. The pelvic thrust, 3 minutes.
5. Third set of jumping squats, 10 repetitions.
6. Pelvic circles, 3 minutes.
7. Fourth set of jumping squats, 10 repetitions.

DO PELVIC RESISTANCE EXERCISE

Resistance exercise basically means moving heavy objects or moving against immovable objects. The testes respond even *more* to resistance exercise than to cardio workouts.

Resistance exercises actually raise your T even more than aerobic exercises. This is partly because muscle is being challenged: when this occurs, the body sends building signals, and the body immediately requisitions more testosterone.

But both types of exercise—cardio and resistance—are important for an integrated health-care plan.

How Much Pelvic Resistance Exercise Should You Do?

Try to do fifteen minutes of pelvic resistance exercise, two to five times per week.

Pelvic Resistance Exercises Work Your Perineal Muscles:

WHEN YOU SIT on a bike, you're sitting on your perineum. That's where some of the muscles are that are being challenged in the pelvic resistance exercises.

If you can do all of the following exercises at a first-class facility, with lots of fancy machines, great.

But often people spend huge amounts of money on machines for the home, or on deluxe club memberships, but they don't use them. And then they ask for a doctor's note to try to get a refund on medical grounds.

Also, don't hide your home equipment. Put your exercise equipment in a prominent place, not hidden in a corner of your home. If you see it, you might use it. Don't use it as furniture, or for draping with clothes. If you find it to boring to use, exercise while watching television or videos, or listening to music or the radio, instead of spending your entertainment time as a couch potato.

PS: If you do put in time at a fitness club already, use the skills detailed here to focus more on the *pelvis.* You need good circulating levels of T for your muscles, bones, blood vessels, and brain to respond optimally to overall fitness training.

Pelvic Thrust, with Weight on Abdomen

1. Lie down as if you're about to do a sit-up: legs bent, knees up, feet on the ground.
2. Place a substantial weight on your lower abdomen. This could be a large book, or a ten-pound dumbbell.
3. Hold the weight steady on your abdomen with your hands.
4. Begin slow, measured, full pelvic thrusts.

The idea here is to feel the full movement. This uses the same principle behind Pilates workouts—do fewer repetitions but maximize the value of each movement.

You need a baseline of five minutes for this exercise. Count time, not the number of repetitions.

Thigh and Pelvic Workouts
You have a number of choices here:

Knees Going Inward
This is for inward thigh movements. You need a large ball. A soccer ball is ideal, or a deflated basketball, or a firm foam exercise ball.

1. While sitting comfortably on the ground or on a chair, place a large ball between your legs, close to the knees.
2. Squeeze inward, using not only your thigh muscles but also recruiting your pelvic and perineal muscles. Use slow, steady, measured contractions.

Some men borrow their wife's Thighmaster equipment to do this.

You need a baseline of three minutes for this exercise. Again, count time, not the number of repetitions.

Knees Going Outward
This is for outward thigh movements. You need a belt, tied or buckled to its maximum size.

1. Sit in a comfortable chair.
2. Wrap the belt tightly around your knees, as if you're bound with rope.
3. Push outward against the belt, feeling not only your thigh muscles but also recruiting your pelvic and perineal muscles. Again, slow, steady, and measured.

Men like this exercise; this is one they can do even at work, sitting at a desk. Some men even take off the belt they have worn to their office to do this, then put it back on when they're done. When asked why, their typical reply is interesting. They'll say, "If I get a belt just for the exercise, I know it will just sit in some drawer and I'll never use it. I won't even remember where it is after a while. This belt [the one they're wearing] reminds me to do the exercise."

You need a baseline of three minutes for this exercise. Again, count time, not the number of repetitions.

A variation of this is: If you have a desk in which your legs can reach the edges of the enclosing drawers, you can push outward against the desk.

Modified Male Kegel Exercises

These exercises were originally developed for women who had problems controlling urination. They have been modified and used for everything from sexual dysfunction and control of the sex act to better orgasms.

Some muscle anatomy: There's a whole group of muscles that hangs down in a big U, like a suspension bridge, from your front pubic bone to the bottom of the tailbone. This bridge has lots of off-ramps, and controls the whole floor of the pelvis. It's where your perineum lives.

Find your access points for the exercise:

1. Tighten your anus, as if you're trying to stop stool from coming out.
2. Tighten your bladder, as if you're trying to stop urine from coming out, or trying to lift your penis up by its own muscle contractions.
3. You will feel a lifting sensation as you do these. Focus on these muscles, as those are the contractions you need to perform together to do this exercise.
4. Now, tighten these muscles in a long, *slow*, steady contraction.

You need to do ten repetitions of ten-second contractions.

> ONE OF THE benefits of modified male Kegels is to delay ejaculation. This prolongs and increases your sensations, and allows for a higher T-release after orgasm.

Flex Gluteals

These are your buttocks muscles, what you sit on. Hold each of these contractions for ten seconds:

1. Slowly and fully contract and release right gluteal.
2. Slowly and fully contract and release left gluteal.
3. Slowly and fully contract and release both gluteals together.

Men like this exercise also, as it's portable. It can be done anywhere—sitting at a meeting, waiting in your car at a stoplight, and so on.

You need a baseline of three minutes for the entire process. Feel the quality of the contractions during your exercise.

Suggested Pelvic Resistance Workout Schedule:
1. Knees going inward, 3 minutes.
2. 1 minute rest.
3. Modified male Kegels, 3 minutes.
4. 1 minute rest.
5. Knees going outward, 3 minutes.
6. 1 minute rest.
7. Flex gluteals, 3 minutes.

A Small Complaint about Being Buff

MEN WHO REGULARLY pump iron or exercise in gyms often have the wrong focus. They think about the their appearance, how good they look, the contour of their body, or their strapping muscles—all external considerations.

Their interest is often to entice someone, for personal vanity, to outdo their peers, and—lastly—to achieve good health.

Men need to spend time exercising their insides, their internal world. Their focus on their upper body should be replaced by a focus on their internal body. That's what the components of the two pelvic regimens detailed here are about. Remember, a tuned, juiced pelvis has more health benefits than bulging biceps or chest muscles.

WHAT YOUR BODY SAYS TO ITSELF WHEN YOU EXERCISE

Exercise affects you in deep ways.

Doing regular exercise tells your body to cater to your needs—by increasing blood supply, turning on protein factories, cleaning the pipes, making sure resources are allocated as necessary. All systems are activated: circulation, hormones, muscles, bones, the genes, and so on. It also sends an important message to your body that you're not giving up, you're still in the game, you still matter, you're in control.

When you perform these exercises, your pelvis is saying, "Okay, I can see that this area of our body is very important to you, so I'll make sure I keep this place juiced, prepped, toned, and ready to burn with T."

But if you do *no* exercise, like six out of ten North American men, your pelvis will say, "Fine, we're not expecting much out of you anymore. We are going to make you less attractive, less upbeat, so that your tired old seed will stay at home and go to the grave."

Don't neglect your pelvis.

> ## Which Order of Exercise Leads to Higher T-Delivery?
>
> 1. (A) Cardio *then* resistance
>
> *or*
>
> 2. (B) Resistance *then* cardio
>
> *Answer: (B) Resistance first.*
>
> If you can do both your resistance and cardio workouts together, do the resistance first.
>
> With resistance exercise, your body is asked to make more T. Testosterone is summoned up and is generated in extra quantities to help build, repair, and sustain you through your straining exercises. Then the cardio workout helps to wash out and disperse that newly created T throughout the bloodstream.

FIDGET

This is especially important for the huge number of North American men who spend their days mostly sitting.

Fidget all the time. Shake your foot, tap your toe, shake your hand, tap a pen, whatever. If you do this persistently, it burns a surprising number of calories. This can be almost as powerful as formal exercise, *if done regularly.*

Having the fidgeting habit can lead to burning off calories worth twenty pounds of fat in one year. This is a remarkable way to incorporate a calorie-burning strategy into your daily routine.

INTERNAL
MEDICINE

5

Background
Questions

YOUR INTERNAL WORLD concerns all the chemical reactions, nutrients, blood vessels, and policing systems that keep you fit, healthy, and vital.

You'll begin your internal assessment with this section. Rate and score yourself. Once again, think of your score rating—Mild, Moderate, or Severe—as how urgently you need to follow the recommendations in part 2. (If you want to know the full story right away, see appendices A, B, and C. But I recommend that you work your way through the book in the chapter order given.)

——— Your Medical Background ———
(14 questions)

1. *Is this you?* "I smoke cigarettes daily."

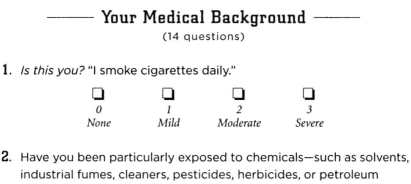

	0	1	2	3
	None	Mild	Moderate	Severe

2. Have you been particularly exposed to chemicals—such as solvents, industrial fumes, cleaners, pesticides, herbicides, or petroleum products?

	0	1	2	3
	None	Mild	Moderate	Severe

3. *Is this you?* "I have had groin hernia(s) and or mumps."

❑	❑	❑	❑
0	*1*	*2*	*3*
None	*Mild*	*Moderate*	*Severe*

4. Do you have a close male relative who died of cancer?

❑	❑	❑	❑
0	*1*	*2*	*3*
None	*Mild*	*Moderate*	*Severe*

5. During your childhood, were you verbally, physically, or sexually abused?

❑	❑	❑	❑
0	*1*	*2*	*3*
None	*Mild*	*Moderate*	*Severe*

6. *Is this you?* "I have been diagnosed with depression at some time in my life."

❑	❑	❑	❑
0	*1*	*2*	*3*
None	*Mild*	*Moderate*	*Severe*

7. *Is this you?* "I am obese, really overweight."

❑	❑	❑	❑
0	*1*	*2*	*3*
None	*Mild*	*Moderate*	*Severe*

8. Do you have a close male relative who had a heart attack?

❑	❑	❑	❑
0	*1*	*2*	*3*
None	*Mild*	*Moderate*	*Severe*

9. *Is this you?* "I have heart disease."

❑	❑	❑	❑
0	*1*	*2*	*3*
None	*Mild*	*Moderate*	*Severe*

10. *Is this you?* "A number of male members of my family have died before age 50."

❑	❑	❑	❑
0	*1*	*2*	*3*
None	*Mild*	*Moderate*	*Severe*

11. *Is this you?* "I have high blood pressure."

❏	❏	❏	❏
0	*1*	*2*	*3*
None	*Mild*	*Moderate*	*Severe*

12. *Is this you?* "I have high cholesterol."

❏	❏	❏	❏
0	*1*	*2*	*3*
None	*Mild*	*Moderate*	*Severe*

13. *Is this you?* "I have sugar diabetes."

❏	❏	❏	❏
0	*1*	*2*	*3*
None	*Mild*	*Moderate*	*Severe*

14. *Is this you?* "Even if I scored very high on this questionnaire, I don't have a health-care practitioner who I feel would really help me.

"My doctor won't take the time to discuss all of my needs, and I don't feel all that comfortable opening up to him, anyway. He might just brush me off by prescribing a sleeping pill or Viagra, or some other drug. He might just tell me to get used to the idea of getting old."

❏	❏	❏	❏
0	*1*	*2*	*3*
None	*Mild*	*Moderate*	*Severe*

Your Medical Background

Your score:_____/ 42 points

Score/Rating
0 to 4   *None*
5 to 17   *Mild*
18 to 34   *Moderate*
35 to 42   *Severe*

Your Habits and Lifestyle

(11 questions)

1. *Is this you?* "I have spent my whole life meeting deadlines."

❏	❏	❏	❏
0	*1*	*2*	*3*
None	*Mild*	*Moderate*	*Severe*

2. Do you have too many late nights?

❏	❏	❏	❏
0	*1*	*2*	*3*
None	*Mild*	*Moderate*	*Severe*

3. *Is this you?* "I do little, if any, exercise."

❏	❏	❏	❏
0	*1*	*2*	*3*
None	*Mild*	*Moderate*	*Severe*

4. *Is this you?* "Over the years, it seems I've devoted too much time and emotion to my work, and not enough to my home life."

❏	❏	❏	❏
0	*1*	*2*	*3*
None	*Mild*	*Moderate*	*Severe*

5. Do you think, "Who has the time to exercise?"

❏	❏	❏	❏
0	*1*	*2*	*3*
None	*Mild*	*Moderate*	*Severe*

6. Do you think, "Who has the time for all those positive, healthy lifestyle changes they keep talking about?"

❏	❏	❏	❏
0	*1*	*2*	*3*
None	*Mild*	*Moderate*	*Severe*

7. Did you have a lot of sexual partners in your life?

❏	❏	❏	❏
0	*1*	*2*	*3*
None	*Mild*	*Moderate*	*Severe*

8. If your wife or partner suggests you get a health checkup, you reply, "Look, I'm fine. There's nothing wrong with me. It'll go away on its own. Let's just forget about it."

☐	☐	☐	☐
0	*1*	*2*	*3*
None	*Mild*	*Moderate*	*Severe*

9. *Is this you?* "I don't have access to good health care."

☐	☐	☐	☐
0	*1*	*2*	*3*
None	*Mild*	*Moderate*	*Severe*

10. *Is this you?* "Yes, sure, I watch a lot of TV. And I spend a lot of time on the computer too, on the Internet. I find it relaxing."

☐	☐	☐	☐
0	*1*	*2*	*3*
None	*Mild*	*Moderate*	*Severe*

11. *Is this you?* "I don't belong to any particular faith. I don't believe in all that religious stuff. There's no higher power, so what's the point of praying? It's just us."

☐	☐	☐	☐
0	*1*	*2*	*3*
None	*Mild*	*Moderate*	*Severe*

Your Habits and Lifestyle

Your score:_____ / 33 points

Score/Rating
0 to 3   *None*
4 to 13   *Mild*
14 to 26   *Moderate*
27 to 33   *Severe*

Consider your score ranges here for the questionnaires Medical Background, and Habits and Lifestyle —did you score None, Mild, Moderate, or Severe? Your scores here will help you determine how urgently you need the recommendations in part 2. These chapters are about diet, heart trouble, obesity, diabetes, supplements, and the genital and urinary systems.

Keep in mind that the suggestions here will help you even if you had good scores, in the None or Mild range. Key preventive health measures discussed here will help to enhance T, even if you are doing well already.

Of course, if you scored in the higher, more problematic ranges—Moderate or Severe, you need these recommendations urgently.

6

Diet

DOES THIS THINKING operate in your household?

- Overfeeding your guests = great hospitality.
- Eating meat = manliness.
- Eating meat = a sign of wealth.
- Being fed = a sign of love and affection.
- Eating rich foods = a sign that you're rich.
- Eating specialty foods = a sign of sophistication.

Food has many meanings and values attached to it. It's about much more than providing healthy fuel for the body—but optimal nutrition should be its primary function. Don't let other considerations interfere with healthy diet choices.

See how you score on this diet questionnaire. Your score will help alert you to food-related concerns.

—— Your Diet ——
11 questions

1. *Is this you?* "I've heard of but don't follow all those 'health' diets; it's all bunk."

□	□	□	□
0	*1*	*2*	*3*
None	*Mild*	*Moderate*	*Severe*

2. *Is this you?* "I pretty well eat whatever I want, whenever I like."

□	□	□	□
0	*1*	*2*	*3*
None	*Mild*	*Moderate*	*Severe*

3. *Is this you?* "I like to snack daily on chips, candies, cookies, or popcorn—just about any munchies."

□	□	□	□
0	*1*	*2*	*3*
None	*Mild*	*Moderate*	*Severe*

4. *Is this you?* "I have more than two alcoholic drinks per day."

□	□	□	□
0	*1*	*2*	*3*
None	*Mild*	*Moderate*	*Severe*

5. *Is this you?* "I have more than two caffeinated drinks per day."

□	□	□	□
0	*1*	*2*	*3*
None	*Mild*	*Moderate*	*Severe*

6. *Is this you?* "I eat a lot of salt."

□	□	□	□
0	*1*	*2*	*3*
None	*Mild*	*Moderate*	*Severe*

7. Is your evening timetable for food and relaxation dictated by the TV program schedule?

□	□	□	□
0	*1*	*2*	*3*
None	*Mild*	*Moderate*	*Severe*

8. *Is this you?* "I don't like the idea of taking pills, and I can't bring myself to take vitamins or supplements regularly."

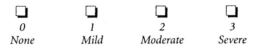

0	1	2	3
None	Mild	Moderate	Severe

9. Do you regularly skip meals, perhaps having only one or two meals per day?

0	1	2	3
None	Mild	Moderate	Severe

10. Do you wonder, "Why does food that's healthy taste so bad, so *blah*? Even a rabbit would get tired of it."

0	1	2	3
None	Mild	Moderate	Severe

11. *Is this you?* "Take care of my nutrition? With the amount of money I spend on junk food, I am personally supporting the fast-food industry. I'm a junk-food junkie."

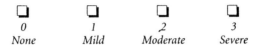

0	1	2	3
None	Mild	Moderate	Severe

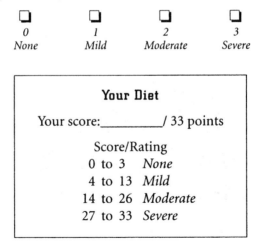

Your Diet

Your score:_____/ 33 points

Score/Rating
0 to 3   *None*
4 to 13   *Mild*
14 to 26   *Moderate*
27 to 33   *Severe*

Consider your score range here—is it None, Mild, Moderate, or Severe? Your score will help you determine how much you may benefit from the recommendations in this chapter. Follow the advice here to benefit from valid and approved dietary recommendations, and to not make poor choices.

NOT EVERY DIET HAS THE SAME GOAL

CLIENTS SAY THAT they can't begin to follow all the various recommended diets, regimens, calorie-counting strategies, food ratings, notions, fads, and prevailing opinions. They are right—I don't blame them. Food recommendations have become too complex, and it seems you need a degree in nutrition science to figure them all out.

These recommendations are powerful, far-reaching, comprehensible, yet relatively straightforward to implement. They are based on these principles:

Key Points

- Your diet should offer revitalizing nutrition and healthy sources of energy.
- Your diet should not wear you down and be unhealthy.
- Your diet should not be merely for taste, comfort, or amusement.
- Much of the North American diet is sludge for the body, toxic to many body systems, including the testosterone system.

These recommendations deal with the quantity and quality of food eaten, additives, hydration, and changing behavior. I make these recommendations to all clients.

Follow each step as best you can. Those with higher scores are advised to follow these suggestions especially closely.

WHAT TO DO

- Eat less.
- *Stop* eating sugar and refined starches as much as possible.
- Reduce salt as much as possible.
- Make water your favorite drink.
- Go easy on caffeine.
- Go easy on alcohol.
- Change from being a meat-and-potatoes man to a seafood-and-vegetables/fruits man.
- Make testosterone-smart choices.
- Avoid fast-food restaurants as much as possible.
- Don't have breakfast on the run and skip meals till dinner.
- Your last meal of the day should be three hours before you sleep.

Ultimately, following these suggestions will benefit your testosterone in some way—either by T-production, release, distribution, effects, or getting rid of T's enemies. This will promote your general health.

EAT LESS

This is the best diet advice you can get.

You may not even realize you are overeating, if your portion is what everyone else is getting too. But the portion sizes served in U.S. restaurants are so large that visitors from other nations cannot believe what one order of food brings.

This supersizing is literally killing us: Portion sizes have grown way beyond our needs and our body's tolerance. For example, a portion of supersize fries has 300 extra calories, compared to regular-size fries. In fact, in a single meal at a resturant, we may unthinkingly consume the caffeine, sugar, and salt intake that's recommended for a couple of days.

One steak house in Texas declares: "$3.99 per ounce. *You* tell us how big." And if you can eat thirty-two ounces in one sitting—that's two pounds—it's free.

Perhaps financially, that's a bargain, but you pay for such overindulgence with your health.

At home, you may also be eating more than a single serving at a sitting. When was the last time you ate only a deck-of-cards-size piece of meat, or the small bowl of cereal considered one portion on the side of the box? By heaping your plate—and consequently overfilling your belly—you may have lost sight of how much food your body actually needs.

Whatever it is that you're eating, *wherever* you're eating, eat less. Don't allow yourself to pig out just because a large portion is available to you.

You *can* cut back without feeling deprived, and without having to carry around a measuring cup and calculator to count calories. Consciously prepare or order smaller portions to begin with, stop eating earlier in your meal than you normally would, and eat slower.

The New Food Pyramid

U.S. FOOD AND Drug Administration recommended daily nutritional guidelines:

Fats, oils, and sweets:	use sparingly
Milk, yogurt, and cheese:	2–3 servings daily
Meat, poultry, fish, dry beans, eggs, and nuts:	2–3 servings daily →

Fruit group: 2–4 servings daily

Vegetable group: 3–5 servings daily

The seven dietary guidelines are:
- Eat a variety of foods to get the calories, protein, vitamins, minerals, and fiber you need for good health.
- Maintain a healthy weight to reduce your chances of having high blood pressure, heart disease, a stroke, certain cancers, and the most common kind of diabetes.
- Choose a diet low in fat, saturated fat, and cholesterol to reduce your risk of heart disease and certain types of cancer. Because fat contains more than twice the calories of an equal amount of carbohydrates or protein, a diet low in fat can help you maintain a healthy weight.
- Choose a diet with plenty of vegetables, fruits, and grain products that provide needed vitamins, minerals, fiber, and complex carbohydrates. They are generally lower in fat.
- Use salt and other forms of sodium only in moderation to help reduce your risk of high blood pressure.
- If you drink alcoholic beverages, do so in moderation. Alcoholic beverages supply calories, but little or no nutrients. Drinking alcohol is also the cause of many health problems and accidents and can lead to addiction.

Source: www.fda.gov

Cutting back on what you eat is easily understood advice. This is important because men generally find it too complex to actually count their calorie intake for any extended period of time.

Eat Less Even if It's a Delicious Meal

"But it was so good. I couldn't really stop."

Let's face it, the more unhealthy a meal is, the better tasting it is. It's these especially appetizing meals that you need to guard against.

Part of the problem is that one truly large meal, or a particularly rich dessert, can neutralize whatever diet control you may have been doing till then. A single huge meal can nullify several days' worth of dieting. So avoid this scenario.

And don't use the excuse, "Sorry, it was a special occasion." There always seems to be a special occasion to use as an excuse for poor food choices.

The 50 Percent Rule

"I'm not sure what's going on. I'm eating the same foods, nothing's changed, but I continue to put on weight."

Observe the 50 percent rule: After age forty, you only need *about half* the food that you ate at age twenty-five.

This halving of the food requirement is startling to most people.

But realize that your metabolism changes with age. If you don't restrict your calorie intake to about half the diet you had in your earlier days, or if you don't burn it off through physical activity, slowly your weight, sugar, cholesterol, blood pressure, and heart attack risk will all increase. If you don't follow this 50 percent rule, you are overloading your system.

Together, all these factors will undermine your health, and drag your T downward.

STOP EATING SUGAR AND REFINED STARCHES AS MUCH AS POSSIBLE

Reducing sugar—and starches that quickly convert to sugar—is a powerful proposal for T-preservation and self-protection. This single recommendation is extremely beneficial and has far-reaching effects.

Some men think we are talking about a polite *reduction* of your sugar intake. We are not—*eliminate* sugar from your diet *altogether*—as close to zero sugar intake as you can.

Certainly, you can count your calories and plan your meals. You can learn about the sugar power of various foods, known as the glycemic index. But men often find this micromanaging of their menu too complex.

Instead of trying to navigate your way through complicated diet recommendations and calculations, it's a lot simpler to stop eating what obviously contains sugar and other simple carbs like highly processed grains.

THE SUGAR FROM natural fruits and fruit juices should be the only sugar that you eat.

To learn more, see the web site www.glycemicindex.com.

Sugar Is Sweet Poison

The extraordinary amount of processed sugar we eat makes it toxic to our bodies over time. This is especially true after you pass the age of forty.

After forty, type-2 diabetes starts to set in, along with many other conditions. This is the time to begin restricting your sugar intake, if you have not already done so.

Eating sugar and other simple carbs every day leads to insulin spikes, which are released to deal with the sugar spikes. This disrupts your entire system, bouncing it between extremes of unnecessary bursts of energy and then fatigue.

On the other hand, men who restrict their sugar intake report that they feel a "calm, steady energy." They are not so easily tired, and they don't crave comfort junk foods.

Sugar also increases the stress hormone cortisol. Together, these factors decrease T-release, and help set the stage for poor health and many diseases.

(See the Diabetes chapter for a full discussion of the effects of sugar.)

Sugar, Sugar, Everywhere

We North Americans eat obscene amounts of sugar—about 150 pounds per person per year. Sugar seems to have become its own food group, on a par with vegetables or dairy products. Clearly, we are overloading our system to the detriment of our health.

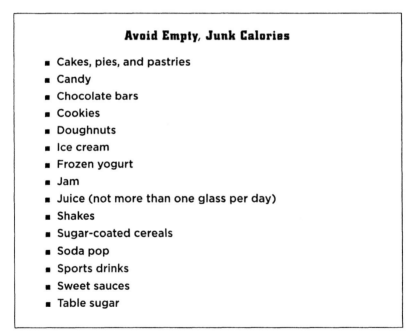

Avoid Empty, Junk Calories

- Cakes, pies, and pastries
- Candy
- Chocolate bars
- Cookies
- Doughnuts
- Ice cream
- Frozen yogurt
- Jam
- Juice (not more than one glass per day)
- Shakes
- Sugar-coated cereals
- Soda pop
- Sports drinks
- Sweet sauces
- Table sugar

You may be trying to control your diet, maybe even exercising reasonably. But with one can of soda pop, which contains about ten to twelve teaspoons of sugar, you can easily neutralize days of diet and exercise efforts. Instead, have *one* eight-ounce glass of *unsweetened* fruit juice every day. (Not grapefruit juice, for reasons discussed on page 76. Also, understand that a juice labeled "no sugar added" does not mean that it is sugar free.)

It is not necessary to end every meal with a baked or dairy dessert. Eat natural, raw fruits as your only source of daily sugar.

Don't Eat Hidden Sugars

Ultimately, simple carbohydrates (starches) are all sugar. Sugar is hiding in these foods:

- Desserts, snacks, and crackers made from refined white flour
- White bread, rolls, and bagels
- White pasta
- White rice
- White potatoes
- High-fructose corn syrup

Do not make any of these sources of hidden sugars part of your daily diet. In fact, a total of twice per week is the limit for these foods. For example, if you have white rice on Monday, and white pasta on Tuesday, do not have any other hidden sugars from this list that week. You have reached your twice-per-week limit.

If you love rice or pasta, switch to brown rice or whole wheat pasta. Eat whole-grain bread products, and switch from ordinary to sweet potatoes (which are a more complex carbohydate, assuming you don't top them with syrup or sugar). Avoid processed foods and condiments that are loaded with corn syrup.

REDUCE SALT AS MUCH AS POSSIBLE

We eat far too much salt.

On average, we eat double the amount of salt that we should—4,000 mg, instead of the recommended limit of 2,000 mg per day. This has a number of health consequences, the major one being high blood pressure.

What Does Excess Salt in Your Diet Actually Do?

Salt makes you retain water in your blood vessels, and retain fluid in the wrong places—in the tissues outside the blood vessels.

To deal with this extra fluid, the heart must pump harder and use more force, squeezing its muscles to accommodate the extra volume.

Ultimately, this can lead to the epidemics of high blood pressure, heart strain, chest pain, heart attack, the need for bypass surgery, stroke, kidney failure, and sudden cardiac death.

These widespread conditions are the reason why doctors have described high blood pressure as a silent killer, a ticking time bomb.

HALF THE MEN in North America die because of cardiovascular causes, either a heart attack or stroke. (A stroke is just a "heart attack of the brain.")

But long before these men die, the same cardiovascular disease processes compromise their testosterone. Two of the cardiovascular consequences of high blood pressure are:

- It deprives the testes of a free-flowing blood supply, both incoming and outgoing. This compromises T production and distribution.
- It contributes to erectile dysfunction.

High blood pressure is quietly damaging people.

Right now, there are about *50 million people* in North America who have high blood pressure. Tragically, half of them do not know that they have it. As they continue to eat excess salt, choosing foods for taste, comfort, or amusement, they don't realize that they are actually eating a cumulative, slow-acting toxin.

Help to defuse this blood pressure bomb, this quiet killer, by drastically cutting back on your salt intake.

Remove the Saltshaker from Your Dining Table

"What can I tell you, doctor? You told him to cut back on salt, but you should see him at restaurants. He just pours it on, like he's making up for lost time. *Shake, shake, shake* . . . and all I can do is shake my head."

The saltshaker on your dining table should become a thing of the past, a relic, like a manual typewriter or reel-to-reel tapes. Don't reach for the saltshaker at restaurants, and it should not be available to you at home. Get rid of it.

Whoever is cooking the meals at home should learn to prepare foods with far less sodium (including baking soda and baking powder). The sodium that comes naturally from actual ingredients (most foods have some) should be the only salt that you are exposed to at home. To add flavor and taste, use salt substitutes, spices, herbs, or simple pepper—none of which generally affect blood pressure.

Beware of fast foods and snack foods, particularly French fries, chips, and pretzels, and sauces, such as steak sauce, which are superloaded with salt. Avoid them as much as possible. Also, be very careful about packaged, processed "low-fat" foods and condiments—many make up for the reduced fat by adding salt, to improve the flavor.

Your Body Will Adjust to the Reduced Salt Intake

"We started the low-salt control. You should see his protests . . . you should see the faces he makes. He complains that he can't taste anything."

When you first start eating a low-salt diet, it will be challenging. Yes, salt adds flavor, making food more appetizing. At first, you may be dismayed by how bland your food has become.

But within a couple of weeks, your body and taste buds will adjust and accept the new low level of salt. You just have to keep at it, and not cheat with a high-salt meal or snack in the meantime.

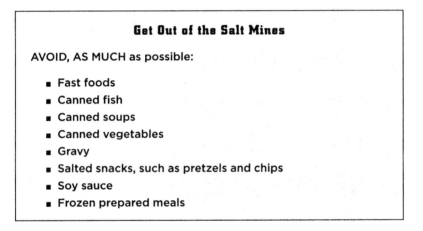

Get Out of the Salt Mines

AVOID, AS MUCH as possible:

- Fast foods
- Canned fish
- Canned soups
- Canned vegetables
- Gravy
- Salted snacks, such as pretzels and chips
- Soy sauce
- Frozen prepared meals

MAKE WATER YOUR FAVORITE DRINK

There are many benefits to drinking adequate amounts of water daily—it's like rinsing your body from the inside.

People seem to know this recommendation, but few follow it regularly.

Drink Six to Eight Eight-Ounce Glasses of Water per Day

Count your intake if you have to; even use a checklist, if it makes it easier. Have a glass or bottle of water near you throughout your day.

The Human Body Is Mostly Water

About 60 percent of the body is water. About 70 percent of the brain is water. So when you drink generous amounts of water daily, you are allowing the body to replace, replenish, and refresh its chief building material.

With proper amounts of water, the electricity in your nerves flows smoothly, you reduce the concentration of toxins, you flush out your toxins, your kidney filters work efficiently, you help keep your joints lubricated, and you have soft stools for easy and complete defecation.

Hydration is also healing—sending extra water is the body's first response to injury. When the body is injured, its first response is to send extra fluid—to swell up, to bathe the affected area, to seal off the injury in a fluid compartment, to create its own sick bay.

In a hospital emergency room, one of the first things we doctors do is give extra fluids to a person by intravenous infusion. We don't wait around for the patient to drink the required amount of extra water, we give it immediately by an IV drip.

You can capitalize on this same hydration-as-healing principle by drinking enough water daily.

Other Fluids Are Not the Same as Water

"I can't drink that much water. Eight glasses? I don't think I need to. . . . Anyway, I get enough coffee or juice and soda. . . . I have about five coffees a day."

Wrong.

Many people do not realize that drinking alcohol, caffeinated beverages, and sugar-laden juices and sodas actually makes you *lose* water. For example, the caffeine in colas, coffee, and tea acts as a diuretic, making you urinate out more fluid than you took in. Generally speaking, you will not be hydrating yourself with most nonwater beverages.

Hydration means drinking *water*.

The Kind of Water You Drink Will Matter over the Long Term

Drink either spring water or bottled water (being careful not to select high-sodium mineral waters).

This may not be easy to do. Both are preferred over tap water. A filtration system for your home water is also recommended as an alternative to buying purified water, and even the simple devices which are attached to faucets, or the pitcher filters, work well.

Where you live determines if your tap water is still reasonable to drink.

The quality of tap water varies greatly across North America. For example, in major cities, tap water has been used and recycled dozens of times, chemically treated for sewage and microbes, chlorinated, and then sent to your home.

The water quality in rural areas is often even poorer. Rural water systems may be polluted—toxins from local industry or farms may have seeped into the groundwater, there may be poor municipal drainage and inadequate water purification, and the faucets, pipes, and plumbing may be ancient, rusted, and decayed.

At the very least, boil and filter your tap water before drinking it.

How Do You Know if You're Drinking Enough Water?

If you are drinking enough water, your urine will be completely clear, colorless, and odorless. This relaxes your kidneys and cardiovascular system, and is proof of water balance, that you are not dehydrated.

Some days you may not have a chance to drink any water or liquids for several hours, perhaps even for the whole day. When this happens, the urine comes out hot, very concentrated, almost burning, possibly with an odor.

This latter situation leads to mild strain on your kidneys and cardiovascular system.

> NOTE: Taking vitamin B supplements can cause orange urine. Beets may turn your urine red. For some people, eating asparagus can cause urine to have a strange aroma. Please discuss with your physician any other unusual colors or odors that continue beyond a bathroom visit or two.

Drink Ice Water

If some of your water intake is ice water, that helps to cool the body.

For optimal function, the testes should stay cool, about 6 degrees Fahrenheit below your own core temperature. Ice water helps to cool your bloodstream ever so slightly, toward that end.

GO EASY ON CAFFEINE

Per day, have no more than two six-ounce coffees, or three caffeinated teas, preferably unsweetened iced tea.

If you regularly drink over these limits, you will diminish your T-release because you will be experiencing the *false* energy of a caffeine rush. Moreover, caffeine is a diuretic, making you actually lose fluid.

Excess caffeine also promotes stomach acid and ulcers, and promotes bone loss.

That Wake-Up Coffee

It is estimated that 90 percent of North American adults have at least one or two caffeinated beverages a day, usually in the morning—to wake up, to focus, to tell their brain that a new day has begun, to be coherent.

> *Can't get going in the morning without a jolt of caffeine?*
> It means you are dependent, and probably addicted to, $C_8H_{10}N_4O_2$—caffeine.

Understand that caffeine is a drug.

Like any drug, it has a measurable dosage—a six-ounce coffee has 100 mg of caffeine. It has its own chemical formula, $C_8H_{10}N_4O_2$. It even has its own appetizing chemical name, 3,7-dihydro-1,3,7-trimethyl-1H-purine-2,6,-dione.

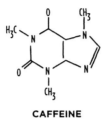

CAFFEINE

And, like some powerful drugs, caffeine is addictive.

However, unlike other drugs, it is not regulated by the Food and Drug Administration (FDA). The only regulation to your dosage is the cup size you prepare at home or order at a coffee shop. A standard-size mug may hold as much as twelve or more ounces of coffee. Likewise, the giant coffees available in specialty shops can hold as much as two days' worth of caffeine—way beyond what you should consume in one sitting.

Consequently, caffeine has become the most widely consumed pharmacological agent in the world. Expecting you to go cold turkey on your morning coffee is unreasonable, but you *can* take measures—literally—steps to control your caffeine intake: by drinking from smaller cups, by mixing decaffeinated and caffeinated coffee to reduce the caffeine level in each cup, or by drinking only decaffeinated and uncaffeinated beverages during the rest of the day.

Want a Hot Drink?

SUBSTITUTE GREEN TEA for tea or coffee. There is emerging evidence that green tea may help prevent cancer.

Don't Live Off the False Energy of Caffeine

Caffeine is a distant cousin of cocaine, and these two drugs have similar effects. Both drugs are stimulants and will rev you up. They will speed up your heart rate, breathing speed, and nerve conduction. They will make you more alert, alter brain wave patterns, release sugar into the bloodstream, increase your blood pressure, and get rid of fatigue.

But this is artificial stimulation.

The problem is that this stimulation is fake—it's false energy. You are tricking your brain to be alert. How? Caffeine elevates levels of the stress hormones cortisol and adrenaline.

Together, these effects diminish the requirement for and output of testosterone. Every time you drink caffeine, your brain–testes axis has to go on a bit of a forced break. Then your body doesn't need so much T for a while. In fact, cortisol and adrenaline dampen and oppose T-output.

A good jolt of caffeine even reduces the blood flow to the brain and the testes. This effect lasts about two to three hours.

Men who drink several coffees a day may feel that they can even do without food for extended periods of time. They're just living off the false, raw, nervous, adrenaline energy of caffeine stimulation.

Your Last Caffeine of the Day

Do not drink any caffeine within two to three hours of your bedtime. If you are particularly sensitive to caffeine, you may need to double this to four to six hours.

As detailed in the Sleep chapter, deep sleep is T-time—the part of the day in which a man's body is bathed in testosterone. Having caffeine close to your bedtime interferes with deep sleep and the nighttime release of T.

GO EASY ON ALCOHOL

Try to limit your alcohol intake to two drinks per day.

Whatever the drink, alcohol is basically sugar and cholesterol—not what you want if you're trying to control your diet. Drinking more than two alcoholic beverages daily is not advisable.

Individuals who regularly drink over these amounts set themselves up for obesity, high blood pressure, heart disease, and diabetes. Why? Chronic, excessive alcohol is a time-released poison for body. It adds too much fat, cholesterol, and sugar calories to the diet. It will slow the amount of fat burned, and will lead to weight gain and a "beer belly."

Alcohol Promotes the Destruction of T

That first drink of alcohol will actually increase your testosterone level. That good feeling you get is part of the temptation to drink.

But alcohol encourages the conversion of testosterone into estrogen, which takes place in abdominal fat cells. Alcohol also acts as a direct irritant to the testes.

After its first rush through your body, alcohol will immediately lower your T production.

In fact, a single episode of getting drunk wipes out about 25 percent of your blood testosterone. The effect lasts for several hours.

This is part of what makes a hangover so bad.

In this way, over time, excess alcohol will diminish T-production and T-effects.

CHANGE FROM BEING A MEAT-AND-POTATOES MAN
TO A SEAFOOD-AND VEGETABLES/FRUITS MAN

Generally speaking, North American men are "meat-and potatoes" kind of guys. This must change for several reasons.

Eating Hormone-Treated Meat Seems to Promote Cancer

Cancer is now the number one killer.

For the first time ever, cancer has overtaken heart disease as the number one killer in North America. This year, 1.5 million people will be newly diagnosed with cancer. The hormones stored in animal fat are part of the reason.

Basically, we are eating the hormones given to animals to enhance meat production and milk output.

Why Use Hormones?

Why would any industry willfully use chemicals that damage people over time? When answering a question of this nature, "follow the money."

Raising animals for meat consumption is more efficient if the animals are treated with hormones. Hormone-treated animals taste better, grow faster, need less feed, give more milk, are heavier, and can be sold for higher prices.

At present, most cattle, lamb, and swine raised for meat consumption in North America are treated with hormones. These chemicals are often given to the animals by implanting slow-release hormone pellets. The hormones leach into the animals' fat cells, and are still there when we consume the meat.

The Chemistry of Your Meat

Hormone enhancers for animals include zeranol (a synthetic estrogen), progesterone, melengestrol (a synthetic progesterone that stops the animals from going into heat), trenbolone (a synthetic half-breed molecule, with both T and estrogen effects), as well as actual testosterone, and estrogen,

It is true that the amounts found in meat as well as milk are tiny, measured in reassuringly miniscule numbers such as nanograms—billionths of a gram. But over time, with a whole generation regularly eating hormone-treated meat, these residues are having biological effects. Estrogen is particularly harmful.

Recently, the U.S. National Toxicology Board listed estrogen as one of the known causes of cancer.

The excess environmental estrogens are also in part responsible for:

- Lower sperm counts in men, a result of T-suppression and T-competition.
- Earlier puberty in adolescent girls—an earlier estrogen debut.

- Increased infertility problems in both women and men. Ironically, hormones given to animals to enhance their fertility are damaging our fertility.
- Increased rates of estrogen-sensitive breast cancers.

North American women are experiencing an alarming increase in breast cancer, which is an estrogen-promoted disease. The rates of breast cancer have been increasing steadily since the 1970s.

Men are experiencing these estrogen effects with diminished T, although they have yet to become conscious of this.

Interestingly, none of these problems is increasing in the third world, where less meat is consumed, and livestock is not treated with enhancing hormones. In fact, sperm counts are *increasing* in non-Western developing nations.

What Is the Government Doing about This?

European Union countries have *banned* the use of hormones to enhance livestock.

The United States, Canada, Australia, Japan, Mexico, and New Zealand continue to allow this practice.

> NOTE: This is not a false alarm, the cry of tree-hugging, pro-Earth, vegetarian, animal rights, antidevelopment, off-the-wall environmental liberal activists *only*.
>
> These hormone effects are real, scientifically documented, and increasing.

We should try to follow the European lead, but there are many challenges. Hormone-treated meat actually tastes better, the agricultural lobby is too strong, and the profits at stake are too large.

Sadly, it may take another generation for government, industry, and the public to admit, understand, and deal with these issues—exactly the time frame it took to wake up to the realities and dangers of cigarette smoking.

> #### Other Environmental Estrogens
>
> THE INDUSTRIAL CHEMICALS used in consumer products are unregulated. We are learning that skin, hair, body, and face products commonly contain chemicals that disrupt hormones.
>
> For example, more than four hundred products contain benzophenone, also known as oxyphenone. This chemical behaves like an estrogenic steroid, and with chronic use can be a hormone disrupter.

Another widely used chemical is phthalate. It has a number of effects, which likely include reducing sperm counts.

Read the labels of your cosmetic and cleansing products, or research their chemical content on such Web sites as the Environmental Working Group, www.ewg.org.

Educate yourself about the many everyday products that may be sabotaging your hormones, and choose products accordingly.

How Much Meat Is Safe to Eat?

Do not eat meat more than twice per week

This includes, beef, lamb, mutton, and pork. These meats should be an occasional treat, not regular staples. When you do have meat, limit yourself to two three-ounce portions per week, which is about the size of a deck of cards or a bar of soap.

Now, this may seem like a tiny serving to you if you are used to eating great slabs of steak or multiple chops in one sitting. But remember that, with each bite, you may be eating more harmful chemicals than you bargained for.

Don't Stop Eating Meat

"Geez, doc. With all those artificial chemicals in it, shouldn't I just stop eating meat altogether?"

No.

I still recommend that you eat meat, although in reduced quantities. In particular, meat has the cholesterol base from which steroid hormones, including testosterone, are made by your own body. A vegetarian diet does not provide you with that.

Also, meat still provides vital components of nutrition, especially protein.

Substitute Poultry for Meat

Though the birds may not have been raised chemical free, among other health benefits chicken, turkey, and other fowl do not have as much animal fat as red meat, and therefore do not store as much hormone. (When eating poultry, remove the fatty layer of skin, to further reduce your fat and chemical consumption.)

Eat Fish Three Times per Week or More

All fish have various benefits, especially sushi, since it's served fresh, and not fried, oversalted, or drowned in creams. But particularly recommended are:

- Anchovies
- Bass
- Crab
- Freshwater trout
- Halibut
- Herring
- Mackerel

- Pollock
- Salmon
- ʻSardines
- Scallops
- Shrimp
- Tuna

ADULT MEN SHOULD restrict their consumption of shark, sword-fish, and fresh and frozen tuna to one meal per week. There is concern about lifetime mercury exposure, particularly in young, pregnant women, who should limit their intake of these fish to one meal per month.

There are a number of benefits from eating generous amounts of fish.

First, when you're eating fish protein, you're not eating beef, lamb, or pork Of course, many restaurants neutralize the benefits of eating fish by offering combo meals that include beef or lamb. Don't order combo dinners. Stick with the fish alone.

Second, many fish are rich in omega-3 fatty acids. These are powerful substances which help to lower blood pressure, reduce cholesterol, and prevent heart attacks.

Eat Fruits and Vegetables Daily

Eat fruits and vegetables daily, at least three servings or more.

The daily number of recommended fruits and vegetable servings keeps going up—from three to five, to as many as nine. Most of the men that we deal with max out at three to four servings a day, which is a reasonable and achievable goal. But the official guidelines recommend:

Fruits: 2 to 4 servings daily.
Vegetables: 3 to 5 servings daily.

Fruits and vegetables help to neutralize processed chemicals; in effect, they are antidotes to the other foods we eat. They offer various vitamins, iron, minerals, water, fiber, and cancer-fighting antioxidants—and all of these together help to neutralize the various toxins that we encounter in meat and processed foods.

People who eat generous helpings of fruits and vegetables daily have less risk of developing cancer. Scientists are noting reduced rates of cancers of the mouth, stomach, colon, bladder, kidney, and ovary. In the same way, men who eat generous helpings of fruits and vegetables daily will fight off estrogen and have enhanced T-effects.

> EATING RAW, FRESH fruits and vegetables delivers more nutrients than eating canned, frozen, or dried vegetables. Choose an array of colorful fruits and vegetables—the more vivid and varied they are, the richer in nutrients.

Choose Green

Green vegetables and fruits contain a number of beneficial plant chemicals—phytochemicals such as lutein and indoles. These function as antioxidants and also help to speed up a number of beneficial chemical reactions. Recommended are:

- Arugula
- Beet greens
- Bok choy
- Brussels sprouts
- Broccoli
- Cabbage
- Cauliflower
- Chicory
- Collard greens
- Green grapes
- Kale
- Mustard greens
- Parsley
- Rapini
- Romaine lettuce
- Spinach
- Swiss chard
- Turnip greens
- Watercress

Choose Orange/Yellow

Orange/yellow vegetables and fruits also contain a number of beneficial plant chemicals—phytochemicals—such as vitamin C, carotenoids, and bioflavonoids. These are being noted for their beneficial effects in preventing heart disease and various cancers, and for keeping the immune system working well. Recommended are:

- Apricots
- Cantaloupe
- Carrots
- Golden raisins
- Lemons
- Mangoes
- Nectarines
- Oranges
- Papaya
- Peaches
- Pears
- Pineapple
- Pumpkin
- Sweet potatoes
- Tangerines
- Yellow pepper
- Winter squash

Choose Red

Red vegetables and fruits contain the phytochemicals known as lycopenes and anthocyanins. These help promote a healthy genital and urinary system, protect against various cancers, and also protect against heart disease. Recommended are:

- Cherries
- Cranberries
- Raspberries
- Red grapes

- Strawberries
- Tomatoes (including juice, paste, sauce, and ketchup)
- Watermelon

Choose Blue/Purple

Blue/purple vegetables and fruits also contain a number of beneficial phytochemicals, such as anthocyanins and phenolics. These also function as antioxidants and are gaining more attention for their antiaging properties. Recommended are:

- Blackberries
- Blueberries
- Eggplant
- Plums

- Prunes
- Purple grapes
- Raisins

Get Enough Fiber

THE FIBER IN vegetables and fruits helps to reduce sugar and cholesterol, which decreases insulin, which in turn enhances T-effects.

Fiber is also present in whole grains: whole wheat, wheat bran, oat bran, oatmeal grain products.

Make Raw Vegetables Your Snack of Choice

If you find yourself needing to munch between meals, during a busy work session, commuting, or while you watch television, have a variety of precut raw vegetables at the ready—broccoli and cauliflower florets, and carrots, celery, cucumber, and zucchini sticks. These can be prepared in advance and refrigerated, then brought along or set out whenever you feel the urge to nibble. Aside from reducing your tendency to reach for junk food, this will help to build up your recommended level of fruits and vegetables.

Rotate your color choices for variety, and experiment.

MAKE TESTOSTERONE-SMART FOOD CHOICES

Don't Be Too Vegetarian

Strict vegetarians may not get enough fat and cholesterol. Steroid hormones, such as T, start with a cholesterol base. So you do need some animal fat in your diet.

Also, strict vegetarians often have low hemoglobin, suffering from iron deficiency anemia. This diminishes the quality of your blood and your T-transport.

Help Your Liver Clear Out Estrogen

The liver is responsible for digesting and clearing the body of estrogen. Certain foods help speed up the liver enzymes that metabolize—eat up—estrogen. These foods include:

- Broccoli
- Cauliflower
- Shellfish
- Oysters

Choose Foods that Slow Down the Aromatase Enzyme

Aromatase is the enzyme found in abdominal fat. It converts T into estrogen. If you diminish the activity of this enzyme, you have more T and less estrogen.

That's what red grapes and their seeds do.

Red grapes and their seeds contain flavonoids, plant chemicals that help to slow aromatase. This is part of the benefit of drinking red wine, and eating red grapes and their seeds.

Avoid Grapefruit

Grapefruit contains chemicals that slow down the liver's breakdown of estrogen. Eating grapefruit allows more estrogen to hang around in the bloodstream to exert its effects. People taking a statin (cholesterol-lowering drug) should not eat grapefruit, as it can intensify the effect of the drug.

Enhance T-Production
Eat Celery

Fresh celery sticks help the T-production cycle. Celery is thought to do this by promoting circulation. Incidentally, celery also helps the body release androsterone, an aphrodisiac found in perspiration as a pheromone.

Eat Oysters

Oysters contain a great deal of zinc, which itself enhances T-production.

Spice It Up

Various spices counteract environmental estrogens, known as xeno-estrogens. Certain spices speed up the liver enzymes that metabolize estrogen, known as the cytochrome p450 enzyme system, so estrogen is cleared from the body more efficiently.

These spices include:

- Cardamom
- Cayenne
- Curry
- Garlic
- Onion
- Turmeric

Use Soy Carefully

Soy, soybeans, soy milk, soy flour, soy-based baby formulas, tofu, and miso all contain phytoestrogens.

The phytoestrogens in soy are about 1/1000 as strong as the real estrogen made by the human body. But they are *still* estrogens.

Male infants fed mostly soy-based formulas are beginning to show delays in testes maturation, lower-weight testes, and reduced sperm production.

Why?

Phytoestrogens oppose T.

How does this translate for adult males?

- If you are overweight, enjoy lots of soy products.
- If you are close to your ideal weight, avoid soy products.

If You Are Overweight

If you are overweight, your body will tend to have its own excess, real estrogen. Eating soy introduces a weaker, imitation estrogen that binds to the same sites as the more powerful human hormone. The phytoestrogens act as a decoy.

In this way, soy phytoestrogens block the stronger, real estrogen from act-ing, help displace the stronger hormone from receptor sites, and stimulate the faster breakdown of all estrogens by the liver. The liver thinks there's so much estrogen coming its way that it revs up its digestive enzyme system.

If you are overweight, eating soy phytoestrogens will benefit you.

If You Are Not Overweight

If you are not overweight, and if you eat a lot of soy, you will be unnec-essarily introducing external estrogens. Those plant estrogens will then compete with your own testosterone, which you don't want. So avoid soy if you are close to your ideal weight.

Be Selective about Oils

Liberally use:

- Olive oil
- Sesame oil
- Canola oil
- Walnut oil

These oils are low in saturated fats, easily digested, and do not block arteries the way other oils do.

Drink Low-Fat Milk

Milk is a good source of protein and calcium. You may not be consuming enough. Many men use only a small amount of milk in their coffee or in breakfast cereal. The current recommendation is that you have one to two eight-ounce glasses of milk per day.

Use only low-fat milk, either 1% or 2%. The lower fat content helps to protect the body from external estrogens, and reduces cholesterol exposure.

AVOID FAST-FOOD RESTAURANTS AS MUCH AS POSSIBLE

I guess it was just too many cheeseburgers.

—Bill Clinton, 2004,
on the eve of his heart bypass surgery.
Mr. Clinton is also the survivor of a second heart operation, in 2005.

Fast food has too many fried items, caffeine, cholesterol, sugar, salt, fat, grease, and trans fats. The typical burger plus fries plus soda violates most of the dietary advice given in this chapter.

If you must go to a fast-food restaurant, try to order salad, chicken or fish (not deep-fried; grilled is better), and ice water.

A Plea to Food Executives

CUTTING BACK ON these convenience foods requires a cultural change. I respectfully ask executives in the food industry who may be reading this to help foster changes for better national health.

Don't just exploit people's weakness for convenience, salt, sugar highs, and tasty but unhealthy grease.

DON'T HAVE BREAKFAST ON THE RUN AND SKIP MEALS TILL DINNER

It's easy to tell men that it's important to have a proper breakfast. But it is a real challenge to get them to adopt this advice in their own lives.

Typically, a North American man will have breakfast on the run—maybe a muffin (which is essentially cake, not even a bread product) and coffee, some toast and jam, or a bagel and cream cheese. And that's it.

Then he will supplement his energy requirement with multiple coffees throughout the day, full of sugar and cream, along with a sweet snack such as a doughnut, pastry, or piece of cake, or another bagel or muffin. Often, there will be no time for lunch, and he will continue to live off the false high of caffeine till dinner.

By then, he'll be really hungry, so dinner will be too large, he'll be too tired to do any physical activity and will just veg out for several hours in front of the TV, and then he'll go to bed.

This is the worst possible schedule you can follow for testosterone.

What Happens When You Skip Meals?

When you have breakfast on the run, multiple coffees, snacks instead of food, and nothing else till a heavy dinner, your body must secrete large quantities of the stress hormones cortisol and adrenaline. This will give you a simulated energy to make it through your day.

If this secretion goes on for several hours all day, that will smash the T-response.

Have a Proper Breakfast, Lunch, and Dinner

Distribute your food intake throughout the day, so that you will have a steady supply of genuine nutrients. This is the idea of smaller meals at spaced intervals. Don't just wing it on coffee and sugary snacks.

A good breakfast choice is a bowl of high-fiber cereal, with no added sugar, with low-fat milk; or low-fat yogurt, fruits, nuts, and peanut butter on brown toast.

Eat a nutrient-rich but modest lunch of chicken or fish, whole grains, vegetables, and fruit. You'll tap into that, rather than need coffee, for your energy until dinnertime, when again you should eat lightly and sensibly.

Once this has become habitual, you'll be surprised by how much more energetic and attentive you'll be throughout the day.

YOUR LAST MEAL OF THE DAY SHOULD BE NO LESS THAN THREE HOURS BEFORE YOU SLEEP

If you eat and then go to bed soon after, your body is still busy digesting its food. The brain is preoccupied with secreting digestive enzymes and acids from the stomach and pancreas. Blood flow is preferentially directed toward your thirty-foot intestine, which does its own aerobic dance workout, moving in a coordinated wave pattern called peristalsis. Insulin levels are still high, dealing with sugars and carbohydrates. And the liver is put on alert to receive digestive breakdown products for further processing and elimination.

This is a demanding process, and lasts about two to three hours after a large meal.

Collectively, all these events diminish testosterone production and distribution, as the brain's focus, blood flow, muscle action, and attention are all directed toward digestion. If you sleep too soon after an evening meal, this will cut into the all-important nightly T-exposure.

7

Heart Trouble

THE WIDOW OF a forty-five-year-old man recalls the day her husband died. "He came home for lunch and said he had a little chest pain. It seemed like nothing, *nothing*... maybe some heartburn. That's all we thought it was. How was I supposed to know that he was having a heart attack? I'm not a doctor... Rob [her husband] had some ice water, said he felt better... then he went back to work. God, can you believe it—back to work? He even *drove* himself.

"Two hours later they called—they found him collapsed in his office. The paramedic guys, well, what were they supposed to do? Robbie was already gone... I still find it hard to deal with. He seemed so healthy, so full of life."

It is said that men suffer from silent diseases—high blood pressure, high cholesterol, undiagnosed diabetes, osteoporosis, and so on.

Doctors wonder, are the diseases silent, or are *the men who get them* silent?

Whatever the case, it's time for men to speak up and for the diseases to be brought out into the open.

All men can benefit by following the suggestions in this chapter, but especially those who had high scores in the Medical Background, Habits and Lifestyle, and Diet questionnaires.

Pay special attention to the Heart Risk questionnaire on page 84.

A Message to All Men over Forty

START TAKING CARE of your heart before you really have to.

HEART DISEASE IS ON THE RISE

ONE MILLION PEOPLE die from heart attacks every year. Robert, a forty-five-year-old computer engineer, was one of them.

Heart disease continues to afflict men in epidemic proportions, and the number of men at risk is staggering:

These are not meaningless statistics. These numbers represent real people: grandfathers, fathers, sons, husbands, uncles, friends, colleagues— maybe even you or your loved one.

- Overweight men are now in the majority.
- Fifty million men have high cholesterol.
- Thirty million men have heart disease right now, with varying degrees of blocked arteries.
- Thirty million men have high blood pressure.
- Ten million men have diabetes right now, with even more scheduled to develop the condition over the next ten years.

Half of all men will suffer the consequences of these risk factors.

Half of all men will die because of cardiovascular disease—by either a heart attack or a stroke. And the proportion is growing.

WHY AREN'T DOCTORS MORE ON TOP OF THIS?

WHEN A MAN over forty sees a doctor, the doctor should size up the client's heart status. Doctors should think to themselves, "Is this client going to be the one out of two men who will have a heart attack or a stroke in the future?

There's a checklist that we doctors ought to go through to get a proper sense of our clients' cardiac risk.

Unfortunately, the vast majority of men who need to have this type of audit do not get it. There are many reasons: men may not have health insurance or a primary care physician, or can't be bothered to see doctors, or don't want to follow their doctor's advice.

In other cases, the doctors are too rushed to give proper time to their clients, or the clients may have come for other reasons that use up all the time. It's also possible that the doctors may not practice preventive medicine—and will only start talking to you about heart disease *after* you develop it.

Gum Disease Is Related to Heart Disease

THE TARTAR AND decay in teeth and gums can lead to heart disease. The germ-laden debris triggers an ongoing immune self-attack.

The body launches this attack to eliminate the bacteria. But it leads to friendly fire against the walls of blood vessels in the heart and elsewhere. This leads to scarring, toughening, and blockage of the vessels.

Over time, that's how gum disease can cause cardiovascular disease.

Keep your heart healthy by seeing your dentist for regular checkups and cleanings.

Key Points
- Cardiovascular disease opposes testosterone.
- Testosterone opposes cardiovascular disease.

CARDIO + VASCULAR = HEART + BLOOD VESSELS

BASICALLY I'M SAYING this—*blood flow equals happiness.*

Blood vessels and blood flow are very important.

If you keep the blood vessels in working order, and the brain and testes get the river running through them that they need, then they'll uphold their end of the bargain. They'll keep you T-loaded. Otherwise they can't.

Blood remains in any one part of the body for less than a second. It keeps getting pulsed away with the heartbeat. Testosterone has to seep into that passing stream in this short time, second to second, beat to beat.

This isn't going to happen if arteries get plugged up. If you let the blood vessels get blocked, and keep eating sludge you call food, what can be done? There's only so much the brain–testes axis can recover from.

Consider the slender testicular arteries, the supply line to the testes. These are only half a millimeter in diameter, about the size of a thick piece of paper.

Hardening of the testicular arteries—atherosclerosis—has many effects. It interferes with the production orders coming from the brain, with the local manufacture of T within the testes themselves, and with the general delivery of T throughout the body.

With narrowed blood vessels, the brain cannot send signals to the testes so easily. Less nutrients arrive. And there is diminished dispersal of testosterone, as the delivery pipes throughout the body steadily get clogged.

Take care of the plumbing, not just for your heart, but for the testes down there, too. All body systems will benefit.

Remember, *Cardiovascular disease opposes testosterone.*

WHAT TO DO

- Take the Heart Risk questionnaire.
- Understand that when your heart system weakens, your testosterone capacity weakens.
- Understand that when your testosterone capacity weakens, your heart system weakens.
- Understand the importance of age forty.
- Test yourself annually to monitor your cardiovascular status—which mirrors your testosterone status.
- Have a firm grasp of what the tests mean.
- Follow the T-strengthening protocols throughout this book.

TAKE THE HEART RISK QUESTIONNAIRE

Just being a man over age forty is *two* risk factors for having a heart attack: gender plus age.

This self-inventory will help to determine if you are at risk for cardiovascular disease. *Please share your responses to this questionnaire, your heart history, with your partner, or with your health-care practitioner.*

——— The Heart Risk Questionnaire ———
(16 questions)

Background

1. Are you a man over 40?

   ❏   ❏
   Yes   *No*

2. Did your grandfather, father, or brother have a heart attack or stroke?

   ❏   ❏
   Yes   *No*

Habits

3. Are you physically inactive?

    ❏   ❏

    Yes   *No*

4. Are you overweight?

    ❏   ❏

    Yes   *No*

5. Do you smoke daily?

    ❏   ❏

    Yes   *No*

6. Do you eat fast foods at least twice a week?

    ❏   ❏

    Yes   *No*

7. Do you eat too much red meat?

    ❏   ❏

    Yes   *No*

8. Is there too much salt in your diet?

    ❏   ❏

    Yes   *No*

9. Are you stressed out a lot?

    ❏   ❏

    Yes   *No*

10. Do you have more than two alcoholic drinks a day?

    ❏   ❏

    Yes   *No*

Conditions

11. Have you had your first heart attack already?

    ❏   ❏

    Yes   *No*

12. Do you have high blood pressure?

    ❏   ❏

    Yes   *No*

13. Do you have high cholesterol?

☐   ☐
Yes   *No*

14. Do you have diabetes?

☐   ☐
Yes   *No*

15. Do you have erection problems?

☐   ☐
Yes   *No*

16. Do you have bad gums that bleed easily when you brush?

☐   ☐
Yes   *No*

From these sixteen questions, total the number of YES answers. This estimates your risk for heart disease.

The two wild cards are these: if you have already had a heart attack, then your arteries—including those going to the testes—are already partially blocked. You automatically go into the Severe risk category.

Also, if you have diabetes, then you also automatically go into the Severe risk category.

Your Heart Attack Risk
Score/Rating
0 to 2   *None*
3 to 5   *Mild*
6 to 10   *Moderate*
11 to 16   *Severe*

Graph your score. For example, if you had 8 Yes answers, you would draw a straight line through the bar graph as shown, the *Moderate* category.

UNDERSTAND THAT WHEN YOUR HEART SYSTEM WEAKENS, YOUR TESTOSTERONE CAPACITY WEAKENS

The heart is the mover of the hormone down the arterial road. So far, doctors have understood this to be a one-way equation:

Cardiovascular		Weakening
Disease	⟶	**Testosterone**

But this cause-and-effect relationship actually goes *both* ways. And this is just beginning to be appreciated by medical science.

The relationship between a good heart and good T levels is direct:

Basically, the pumping heart and clean blood pipes are the courier system of the testes, required for incoming raw materials, and for outgoing finished product.

Testosterone builds and keeps heart muscle strong. In fact, there are more T receptors in the heart—waiting to be juiced—than in any other muscle of the body.

However, the same factors that put men at risk for cardiovascular disease also put them at risk for weakening testosterone. The risk factors for one are the risk factors for the other. Poor circulation leads to both.

High cholesterol, high sugar, high blood pressure, high stress, lack of physical activity, and obesity all oppose T.

The processes that cause arterial blockages also cause lower amounts of T, and poorer delivery of T to body tissues.

UNDERSTAND THAT WHEN YOUR TESTOSTERONE CAPACITY WEAKENS, YOUR HEART SYSTEM WEAKENS

Doctors can sense that a weakening cardiovascular system leads to weakening T. But when you examine this relationship closely, it also becomes clear that *weakening T leads to a weakening cardiovascular system.*

This is a revolution in thinking: T deficiency leads to heart disease.

Weakening T contributes to high cholesterol, high sugar, high blood pressure, high stress, a reluctance to do physical activity, and obesity. Weakening T is one of the initial *causes*, the initial *triggers*, of all of these conditions.

The cumulative effect of this is that a man with weak testosterone will lose up to 25 percent of the blood flow to his heart.

So, the equation goes the other way too:

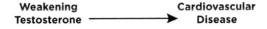

Weakening		Cardiovascular
Testosterone	⟶	**Disease**

This has massive implications: you can help your heart and blood vessel system *by building T.*

Cardiovascular Disease and ED

Erectile dysfunction is a common example of this interplay between cardiovascular disease and weakening T.

In this condition, the cause-and-effect equation plays out both ways simultaneously, in a self-reinforcing cycle:

```
Weakening    ──────────▶  Cardiovascular
Testosterone ◀──────────      Disease
```

For an erection, about six times the normal amount of blood must flow into the penis. A man with the various cardiac risk factors has a high chance of having erection problems. This will lead to less sex, less pleasurable orgasms, less desire, fewer T storms, and less T distribution. The reduction in T will accelerate and accentuate cardiac problems, which will lead to less sex, less pleasurable orgasms, less desire, fewer T storms, and less T distribution.

And so the cycle continues.

Doctors are only now being taught to think of erection problems as an early warning, a signal, of heart disease.

If you have erection problems, you have a 20 to 40 percent chance of also having heart disease. And if you have heart disease, you have an equally strong chance of having erection problems.

UNDERSTAND THE IMPORTANCE OF AGE FORTY

For men, age forty is the launching pad for cardiovascular disease and all its consequences. (For women, it's age fifty that is the turning point.)

Men must pay special attention to their health when they enter their forties, especially if they had never bothered to do so before. Men are able to get away with most things till then—drinking, smoking, lack of sleep, substance abuse, too much stress, minimal exercise, poor diet, excess weight, and frequent sport sex. But now it's payback time—when their body calls in credit that it extended to them in their youth.

The Big Four-Oh Is Inching Up

SO FAR, DOCTORS have used age forty as the cutoff, the time of life after which cardiovascular conditions truly accelerate.

But men seem to be developing cardiovascular problems even

---

earlier. If present trends continue, we may have to lower this cut-off age to thirty-five.

Despite all the advances in medicine and our growing knowledge of what constitutes a healthy lifestyle, modern man is experiencing increasing stresses, poorer eating habits, more accessible substance abuse or casual sex, less physical fitness, and a rise in obesity. The many risk factors and conditions that spring up after forty—high cholesterol, high sugar, high blood pressure, high stress, lack of physical activity, weight gain, heart attacks, chest pain, erection problems, sudden cardiac death, and weakening T are happening sooner. All these illnesses are starting sooner, and this is no coincidence.

If you are not yet forty, don't use the intervening years to abuse your health—you're sure to pay for it, and probably sooner rather than later.

TESTOSTERONE OPPOSES CARDIOVASCULAR DISEASE

After age forty, it is vitally important for a man to mobilize his T as best he can. This will prevent, slow, stop, reverse, or eliminate cardiovascular challenges.

Testosterone increases the body's chemicals that open up blood vessels—nitrous oxide, for example. (That's how Viagra works.) The benefits of fully mobilized and sustained T include:

- Better blood flow everywhere
- Blood vessels that expand more easily, increasing flow on demand
- Less heart pain (angina)
- Better exercise tolerance
- Better utilization of oxygen
- Lower blood pressure
- Redder blood (with more oxygen-carrying hemoglobin)
- More of the "good" HDL cholesterol
- Less of the "bad" LDL cholesterol (the one that sticks and plugs up arteries)
- Fewer blood clot particles (such as fibrinogen)
- Better tolerance of emotional stress
- More drive
- More energy
- More ambition

> Cardiovascular status = Testosterone status.

TEST YOURSELF ANNUALLY TO MONITOR YOUR CARDIOVASCULAR STATUS—WHICH MIRRORS YOUR TESTOSTERONE STATUS

A man's heart will pulse:

- In one year, 37 million times
- In eighty years of life, 3 billion times

That's extraordinary. All aspects of your life depend on keeping your heart working well.

These are concrete medical tests that you should do to track your heart and blood vessel status from year to year:

- Physical Tests
  - Blood pressure
  - Weight
  - Waist measurement
- Electrical Test
  - EKG
- Blood Tests
  - Total cholesterol
  - LDL cholesterol
  - HDL cholesterol
  - Triglycerides
  - Hemoglobin A1c
  - High-sensitivity C-Reactive Protein
  - Homocysteine

HAVE A FIRM GRASP OF WHAT THE TESTS MEAN

Blood pressure (measured in mm, millimeters of mercury)

Your blood pressure should be 120/80 or less.

This is considered the *new* optimal pressure, which is a radical shift in medical recommendations. Most physicians practicing today are still adjusting their thinking to this newly lowered number. Generally, we were taught that only 140/90 or above is high.

Also, everything now has a pre- stage; for example, prediabetes. Prehypertension is between 120/80 and 140/90. For example, 130/85 is now considered prehypertension—high blood pressure in training.

To achieve optimal numbers like 120/80, men will have to follow a number of protocols, particularly a low-salt diet.

Start Measuring Your Blood Pressure with a Home Monitor

The machine you purchase should be digital and should have a properly sized arm-cuff (not a wrist-cuff) that self-inflates automatically.

How often should you measure your pressure? If there are no problems, perhaps once a month is enough. It should be more frequent if you discover a high blood pressure tendency. Also, write the numbers down to show your health-care practitioner.

Do *not* rely on machines that measure blood pressure from the wrist or fingers, or ones found in shopping malls or pharmacies.

What Does High Blood Pressure Actually Do?

HIGH BLOOD PRESSURE hardens arteries, which make them lose their supple elastic recoil. This recoil is needed to give an extra push to distribute blood out of large arteries into smaller, microscopic vessels.

High blood pressure also narrows arteries by packing cholesterol, cells, and clotting materials firmly into the walls.

High blood pressure also pounds at the artery walls, especially where arteries turn right or left or curve. These turning points are areas of high-velocity turbulence, and are often the sites of blockages. These shear forces damage the inner lining of vessels. This can cause vessels to ooze, rip, burst at a point location, or completely explode.

Weight

You need to be as close to your ideal weight as possible. See the chapter on Obesity.

Waist Measurement

If your waist is more than forty inches, you are at high risk for hypertension, diabetes, and syndrome X.

See the chapter on Obesity.

EKG (Electrocardiogram)

This is a tracing of the heart's electrical activity. It is not a perfect test, but it will alert doctors to heart strain, if areas of the heart are not receiving enough blood, if the heart is enlarged because of unrecognized hypertension, or if there is a rhythm disturbance.

Total Cholesterol, LDL Cholesterol, HDL Cholesterol

LDL cholesterol is the "bad," artery-plugging cholesterol. Every couple of years or so national societies keep lowering what they think the optimal LDL value should be. This has been going on for almost two decades.

For LDL, 100 mg/dl (milligrams per deciliter) the current goal, but I encourage my clients to get the number even lower, to 80 mg/dl. This extra aggressive approach helps to *prevent, slow, stop, reverse, or eliminate cardiovascular challenges.*

HDL cholesterol is the "good" brother, responsible for helping to remove cholesterol from arterial walls and preparing it for disposal.

Doctors have been settling for HDL numbers such as 41, 51, or 55 mg/dl. Clients do best with HDL numbers above 60 mg/dl.

Total cholesterol should be *less than* 200 mg/dl.
LDL cholesterol should be *less than* 100 mg/dl.
HDL cholesterol should be *above* 60 mg/dl.

> **Be honest with yourself.**
> If you can't make the lifestyle changes to reach these cholesterol targets, you may have to consider taking prescription cholesterol-lowering drugs, the statins, of which Lipitor and Zocor have had the most success.
> Don't ignore your test results and hope nothing happens. Your cholesterol numbers are too important to leave to chance.

Triglycerides

Triglycerides are also blood fats, the poor cousin of cholesterol. Because they don't get as much attention as cholesterol, doctors and the public are tolerating much higher numbers than they should.

Your triglyceride count should be less than 150 mg/dl (milligrams/deciliter). See the chapter on Diabetes.

Hemoglobin A1c

This essential and powerful test measures how much glucose has been in your blood for the last three months. This is a more accurate test than the finger-prick glucose test, which only measures how much sugar you have at that exact moment.

Your test result should be less than 6 percent.
Doctors should be using this test more.
See the chapter on Diabetes.

High-Sensitivity C-Reactive Protein (hsC-RP)

Interpreted correctly, this is a powerful marker of cardiovascuar risk—the chance of having heart attacks, strokes, and whether a person will survive them. It measures the ambient level of inflammation and immune self-attack—the friendly fire going on in the bloodstream. (But if a person has, say, an obvious infection, this result will be artificially elevated, and is then not a reflection of heart risk.)

Lab values will vary, so you must compare yourself against the laboratory's own reference ranges. For example, some labs report as follows:

RISK FOR HEART ATTACK	HS C-RP RESULT
Low risk	less than 1.0 mg/L (milligrams/liter)
Average risk	1.0 to 3.0 mg/L
High risk	greater than 3.0 mg/L

Doctors themselves are just beginning to appreciate the value of this sensitive marker, which seems to be a *better* predicter of heart attack risk than cholesterol itself.

Homocysteine

This is an amino acid in the bloodstream that predicts cardiovascular risk. Measuring homocysteine levels contributes to the overall risk assessment picture.

In particular, it seems to capture some of the family contribution, the genetic tendency in first-degree relatives to have heart conditions. It's remarkable to be able to measure that in a simple blood test. This test adds information beyond the standard risk factors that we usually focus on, such as cholesterol and hypertension.

This is important because half the men who come to emergency rooms with heart attacks have *normal* cholesterol values. *This means that there is much more to having a heart attack than how much cholesterol you have.*

So doctors must measure risk components other than cholesterol—because cholesterol does not explain half the heart attacks in North America. Homocysteine measurements capture some of that risk.

Lab values vary, so you must compare yourself against the laboratory's own reference ranges. For example, some labs report as follows:

RISK FOR HEART ATTACK	HOMOCYSTEINE RESULT
Average risk	5 to 15 μU/ml (micromoles/milliliter)
Above average risk	15 to 30 μU/ml
High risk	30 to 100 μU/ml
Very high risk	greater than 100 μU/ml

> **"How could I have a heart attack? My cholesterol is normal."**
>
> Half of all heart attacks happen to men whose cholesterol is normal. There's more going on than just cholesterol, more that goes into the making of a heart attack. That's why other tests are important to get a full picture of your cardiac risk.

Assembling all this information helps doctors to determine your current cardiovascular status and likely future course. This gives us deep insight into your T capacity.

These test results are powerful and essential information for all men over forty to have. Men should repeat these tests annually.

FOLLOW T-STRENGTHENING PROTOCOLS

Closely follow the T-strengthening protocols throughout the book to help you achieve optimal cardiovascular numbers, particularly:

- Chapter 2 Sleep
- Chapter 4 Exercise
- Chapter 6 Diet
- Chapter 10 Supplements
- Chapter 13 Stress Levels
- Chapter 14 Therapeutic Self-Massage

8

Obesity

A FOUR-YEAR-OLD asks, "Daddy, what's in your big fat tummy?" All men need to pay attention to their weight.

All men can benefit by understanding the points in this chapter, but especially those who had high scores in the Changing Body, Medical Background, and Habits and Lifestyle questionnaires.

Why Do Men Become Overweight?

We eat too much rich, sugar-laden, oily, or greasy food.

We don't walk much.

We don't exercise much.

We eat too much junk, convenience, snack, or comfort food.

We are growing oversized or supersized, like the portions served to us.

We may even inherit obese genes.

We don't realize that we can mobilize T to help with weight control.

Overweight men are steadily damaging their chemical profiles. The more overweight you are, the more you drag down your T levels, and interfere with your T-responsiveness.

More than 50 percent of all men are overweight. Two out of five men—fully 40 percent—are overweight to the point of obesity, and about 5 percent of men are "morbidly" obese, which means they're more than one hundred pounds above their ideal weight. As a society, it's time we practiced girth control.

Key Points

- Being overweight opposes testosterone.
- Testosterone opposes being overweight.
- Catering specifically to your testosterone helps you to avoid weight gain.
- Catering specifically to your testosterone helps you to lose weight.

WHAT TO DO

- Know your current weight and your ideal weight.
- Understand the key issues.
- Increase your T-rushes to help fight fat.

KNOW YOUR CURRENT WEIGHT AND YOUR IDEAL WEIGHT

How tall you are determines what your ideal weight should be. The following list gives you your maximum ideal weight for your height.

See where you stand. Are you above your maximum ideal weight? If so, then you are, like the majority of North American men, overweight or possibly even obese. For example, if you are 5'9" tall, your *maximum* ideal weight is 169 pounds. If you weigh 185 pounds, you are overweight.

Men are obese when they are about 20 percent (more than 25–30 pounds) above their ideal body weight. If you are 5'9" tall and weigh more than 203 pounds, you are not only overweight but obese.

Height and *Maximum* Ideal Weight and Obesity Start Points

HEIGHT	IDEAL WEIGHT (LBS)	OBESITY STARTS AT (LBS)
5 ft	128	153
5 ft 1	132	158
5 ft 2	136	164
5 ft 3	141	169
5 ft 4	145	174
5 ft 5	150	180
5 ft 6	155	186
5 ft 7	159	191
5 ft 8	164	197

HEIGHT	IDEAL WEIGHT (LBS)	OBESITY STARTS AT (LBS)
5 ft 9	169	203
5 ft 10	174	207
5 ft 11	179	215
6 ft	184	221
6 ft 1	189	227
6 ft 2	194	233
6 ft 3	200	240
6 ft 4	205	246
6 ft 5	211	253
6 ft 6	216	260

Men usually sense when they are overweight. But many of them are startled when they use the tables to learn exactly how overweight they are.

For example, doctors are seeing more and more midlife men who are 40, 50, 70, even 100 pounds above their ideal weight.

Occasionally we even have to say, "We're sorry, sir, but right now you are two people. You are double your ideal weight."

The full range of height and weight distributions can be seen in this graph:

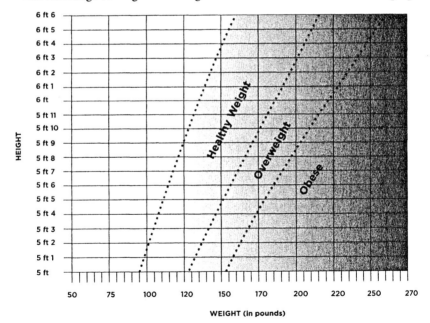

So What's a Pound or Two of Fat?

ONE POUND OF fat adds *two hundred miles* of blood vessels to your body. Being only twenty pounds overweight adds *four thousand miles* of them. And, the more you weigh, the more those extra vessels are clogged with fat.

Your heart has to work harder to move your blood through all those unnecessary pipes—through unfamiliar winding roads, slow-moving traffic, and lots of resistance from the plugging and crusting of the tubing.

This is one of the reasons that extra fat predisposes you to high blood pressure.

Quick Test: Is Your Waist More than Forty Inches in Circumference?

This is a simple test which seems to have the same predictive power as other, more expensive examinations.

Accurately measure your waist using a tape measure placed just above the top of your hip bones.

Don't cheat by sucking in your stomach too much. Exhale first, relax, then measure yourself.

If your waist is forty inches or more, you are at high risk for declining testosterone, cancer, diabetes, heart disease, high blood pressure, stroke, and weak bones, known as osteoporosis.

Toxic Fat:

FAT COLLECTED IN the abdomen is worse than fat elsewhere, for example in the hips, thighs, or legs.

Abdominal fat is chemically very active. For a man, this is nasty, high-risk fat.

UNDERSTAND THE KEY ISSUES

Middle-Age spread

"I haven't changed my eating habits much. I'm doing the same exercise as before. But I keep putting on weight."

Getting a belly?

Have you wondered where your belly came from? In your early forties, did you develop noticeable abdominal fat, a midsection bulge?

If you did not change your diet or exercise levels, you would have gained midsection fat in midlife. This happens to the majority of men in North

America, and they're not sure why. Most men just write this off, without any clear understanding of what's going on. They think, "Well, I must be getting old . . . maybe I'm slowing down a bit." This is true, but they don't understand the underlying chemical basis.

The declining impact of testosterone is the *leading* step that sets off the chain reaction. This is often the first taste of life over forty.

Consider this—the testes are centrally located in front of the body, and the fat deposition in men is also front and center. In essence, the abdomen is testosterone's ghetto.

In women, on the other hand, the ovaries are somewhat to the sides, so a woman's fat gets stored preferentially on the sides—on the hips, thighs, and buttocks.

This is known as gender-specific regional fat distribution.

With declining T, you have less thermogenesis (heat production). You will:

- Burn less energy because of a slower metabolic rate
- Not fight off fatty foods as well as you used to
- Not fight off sugary foods as well as you used to
- Gain weight more easily
- Not be able to lose weight as easily
- Feel like exercising less
- Feel tired more easily
- Not see as good results from exercise
- Have less endurance
- Lose about one pound of muscle every two years—that's huge—mostly from your legs
- Find that the muscle is being replaced by fat
- Feel like you want to take on fewer challenges

With declining T, basically fat replaces muscle.

Being Overweight Turns Your Testosterone into Estrogen
This is shocking, like a chemical kidnapping.

First of all, changing testosterone into estrogen is remarkably easy. The chemical change is very small. It takes one step, a single enzyme, and that's it.

It's like changing the fruit topping on a cake—a trivial thing for the body:

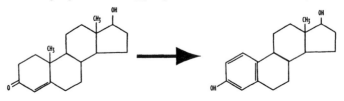

TESTOSTERONE   ESTROGEN

You can barely tell the chemical difference.

Now, the chemistry may not mean much to you, but the simplicity of this conversion is unsettling. It actually seems like a design flaw—to think that the hormone that is the foundation of manhood could so easily lose its character.

What's astonishing is that a first-rate prized product of the man's system, of his testes, the testosterone itself, ordered by the brain, should allow itself to be changed beyond factory specifications so easily by an unrespectable operator such as fat cells.

Truly, this is identity theft and copyright infringement.

Let's walk through the process. The body lovingly makes all this testosterone for you, this superhormone. And what happens? Your stomach fat turns T into estrogen, the woman's hormone. And as stomach fat makes this estrogen, the estrogen tells the fat cells to make *more* of the converting enzyme. This enzyme, aromatase, gets revved up, and then you get even *more* estrogen, in a self-reinforcing cycle.

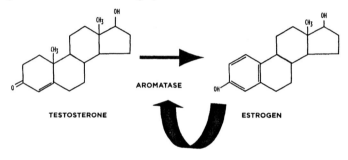

What's more, your abdominal fat is a storage depot, stockpiling and releasing estrogen as it likes. Yet the body can't store testosterone, anywhere. *T can't even be stored in the testes themselves.*

And, to add insult to injury, the chemical reaction only goes one way. T turns into estrogen, but estrogen *cannot* be turned back into T. *This is remarkable and rare for the human body.* Unlike almost all conversion reactions in the body, this is an irreversible reaction, a one-way transaction.

In essence, for a man, having a potbelly is like having ovaries. That's definitely not what you want. *Turning into the enemy.*

Usually, chemical reactions in the body can be reversed:

Amino acids form to make proteins. Proteins can be broken down into their constituents, amino acids.

Cholesterol and fatty acids get stored as fat. Fat can be broken down into its constituents, fatty acids and cholesterol.

> Calcium and minerals solidify into bone. Bone can be broken down into calcium and minerals.
>
> Simple sugars can be stored as glycogen. Glycogen, the storage form of sugar, can be broken down into simple sugars.
>
> But estrogen *cannot* be turned back into testosterone.

And remember, this means testosterone is not just neutralized, burned off, degraded, or eaten up in this reaction. It actually turns into estrogen, the female hormone, that opposes T-effects.

It is remarkable that such a miniscule chemical change, which can lead to such massive physical and psychological effects, is allowed. More and more, this molecular change will stall, diminish, oppose, reduce, or make the body *ignore* a man's T-releases. And slowly it will bring forth, step by step, more of the symptoms highlighted in the questionnaires.

Fat Stores Estrogen

FAT NOT ONLY makes estrogen, it loads up on it, too, storing it away to be released later.

Testosterone cannot be stored anywhere, not in fat, not even in the testes. Nowhere.

It's as if the body thinks T is too powerful, too intense, to be stockpiled anywhere. This is why T is made continuously, and why it responds to current circumstances in real time.

Estrogen Beats Out Testosterone

An overweight man is manufacturing, storing, and releasing enemy estrogen. And when both T and estrogen show up somewhere in the body to exert their respective hormonal effect, estrogen dominates. When estrogen and testosterone compete for receptor sites, estrogen wins. In fact, estrogen actually displaces T.

Their chemical similarity tricks the body.

Because estrogen and T are so chemically similar, almost identical twins, they often act upon the same tissues. They stay at the same hotel rooms, stopping in the same guest spots.

If they both present themselves for the same room, for the same receptor, testosterone foolishly plays the gentleman, and lets estrogen bind to the receptor site. T lets estrogen take the room.

Testosterone is not allowed to sleep on the couch, or even hang around. He is just dispatched without ceremony. By getting the room, occupying the receptor site, estrogen exerts its biological effect.

In this competition, all over your body, estrogen overwhelms testosterone.

If a man wants to have female breasts:

Let yourself get obese, a good 40 pounds or more above your ideal weight is preferred.

Then drink too much alcohol, as this speeds up the aromatase enzyme that converts T to estrogen. Alcohol will also damage the liver, so that estrogen is not digested and cleared away so well, which is the liver's job.

Slowly but surely, you will actually start getting female-type breasts. You don't just get fat *male* breasts. The man's breast tissues start taking on the density characteristics of women's breasts. What's more, this puts men at added risk for breast cancer, usually a woman's problem.

Doctors call this feminization of male breasts *gynecomastia*. That's estrogenization.

The chemical similarity between T and estrogen tricks the brain too.

Since the chemical structure of T and estrogen are so similar, even the brain is fooled. The brain doesn't check the molecular ID thoroughly enough, mistakes estrogen for T, and sends signals to the testes to slow down manufacturing any more testosterone.

Slowly but surely, T-effects diminish *over years*. This leads to the estrogenization of men. The changes are subtle, and that's why men may not recognize these shifts on a day-to-day basis. This is happening right now to varying degrees in more than half the men in North America.

A Major Discovery: Fat Cells Talk *Directly* to the Testes

LEPTINS ARE PROTEINS made by fat cells.

Fat cells make confession through leptins. Fat cells say, "Yes, things are getting too fat around here. Leptins, would you please go ask the testes to secrete more T, to help deal with this obesity."

The leptins then recruit testosterone to help reduce fat. Very unusually, there are leptin receptors in the testes, which were thought to live aloof, in a pure, gated community.

> But when a man is too fat, the leptins can't do their work. Less T is recruited. And the result is increasing food storage, less fat burning, less burning of energy, and less summoning of testosterone to help with weight loss.
>
> Excess weight then overwhelms both leptins and testosterone.

Testosterone Opposes Being Fat

Doctors in Britain are successfully treating potbellies by giving men synthetic testosterone.

The headlines were, "Banish the Beer Belly."

However, this procedure is something I cannot recommend. This can be accomplished with the body's own resources, but the British experience makes the point about the direct relationship between obesity and T. In fact:

Catering specifically to your testosterone helps you to avoid weight gain.

Catering specifically to your testosterone helps you to lose weight.

Men on weight loss programs cater to their T-release without even realizing that's what they are doing. When they control their diet, avoid carbohydrates, do muscle-building exercise, or do cardiac workouts, they are unknowingly enhancing their T-status.

For example, they may feel better after exercise, but they're not sure why. They may have some vague notion that onboard pleasure chemicals, the endorphins, are released after workouts.

In fact, testosterone acts directly on brain cells, and is part of the chemical team that helps set those endorphins off.

Direct and specific T-enhancement bolsters weight management.

INCREASE YOUR T-RUSHES TO FIGHT FAT

Without adequate T, weight-loss strategies won't work. Keeping your T up:

- Helps you to avoid obesity
- Helps you to get rid of obesity
- Helps to speed up your weight-loss strategies

Even modest weight loss helps.

Even a five- or ten-pound reduction is better than none. A five-pound loss takes one thousand miles of unwanted extra blood vessels with it; losing ten pounds removes two thousand miles. Your heart, and the rest of you, will be grateful.

Lose Weight Making Full Use of T-Chemistry
Follow these chapters closely:

- Chapter 2 Sleep
- Chapter 4 Exercise
- Chapter 6 Diet
- Chapter 9 Diabetes
- Chapter 10 Supplements
- Chapter 14 Therapeutic Self-Massage

Even Sleep Helps with Weight Loss

Strangely, we know that men who sleep better lose weight faster. Typical of sensationalist reporting, the press misrepresented this as, "Lose weight by sleeping more." And that, of course, seems bizarre. How could you lose weight by spending more time in bed?

The real story is this: If you have good, restful sleep—more *high-quality* sleep—you get a better, longer, and purer exposure to testosterone. That's what helps with your weight loss. It's the quality, not the quantity, of sleep that matters.

Sleep is T-time.

What If You Have Been Obese Since Childhood?

OVERWEIGHT AND OBESE boys have a downward drag on their testosterone from their earliest days. They miss out on their full T-rushes. This will affect their quality of life, and will shorten their life span as a result.

In such individuals, life expectancy has declined for the first time in North America in two hundred years. The decline was only by a few months, but it was an entirely unexpected change in the usually upward trend of modern man.

Doctors are beginning to see a whole generation of obese men with even lower sperm counts, who set themselves up for many conditions early—declining T, heart disease, diabetes, high blood pressure, and osteoporosis.

There is a comparable problem in obese girls. Such girls are having puberty much earlier, almost three to four years earlier than their mother's generation. The excess estrogen produced in fat will also lead to more fertility problems and higher rates of breast cancer.

About one in three children in North America is now overweight, and the number continues to increase.

9

Diabetes

"Yes, it's been getting annoying. I have to urinate so often during the day . . . I feel thirsty all the time. I thought I was overworked, but something's going on. I'm constantly tired."

All men can benefit by following the suggestions in this chapter, but especially those who had high scores in the Medical Background, Habits and Lifestyle, and Diet questionnaires.

Pay special attention to the diabetes-risk questionnaire below. Important recommendations follow, even if you don't have diabetes (yet).

A Message to All Men over Forty:

STOP EATING SUGAR, as much as possible.

Clients with diabetes have excess sugar floating around in the bloodstream. This leads to many complications, including heart disease, kidney damage, eye damage, nerve damage, infections that don't go away, and possible amputations.

To work well, the brain–testes axis needs the environment to be just right. Then T can be made efficiently, the need for T can be met, and T can be transported quickly. Then T is respected, not ignored, and is used efficiently everywhere.

But it's difficult for that axis to work well in diabetic or prediabetic conditions. If your blood is full of sugar, it's like pancake syrup. Then T production and transport become more difficult, and none of the body's systems function properly.

On top of that, if you are obese, that will itself neutralize testosterone's effects throughout the body.

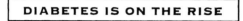

DIABETES IS ON THE RISE

TEN MILLION MEN in North America have diabetes right now. Diabetes is everywhere. It's occurring in epidemic proportions and increasing.

Half of the 10 million men who have diabetes do not know it. They are allowing the disease to damage multiple organ systems in ignorance and silence.

Even more men are en route to developing diabetes.

Another *20 million men* have prediabetes, or diabetes-in-waiting. They will develop the full condition within the next decade.

This is a tragedy and can be prevented. Don't be among the million people who are newly diagnosed with diabetes every year.

The Effect of Diabetes on Testosterone

DIABETES RESULTS IN
- Less T
- Less effective T
- Less distributed T
- Ignored T

Key Points
- Diabetes opposes testosterone.
- Testosterone opposes diabetes.

Once you are prediabetic or diabetic, it's a challenge to have optimal testosterone effects. That's because diabetes dampens, stomps on, and discourages testosterone.

WHAT TO DO

- Take the Diabetes-Risk questionnaire.
- Understand the key issues.
- If you already have diabetes, control it.

- If you don't already have diabetes, avoid developing it.
- Monitor your diabetes potential by getting screening tests annually.
- Reduce your chance of developing syndrome X and diabetes.

TAKE THE DIABETES-RISK QUESTIONNAIRE

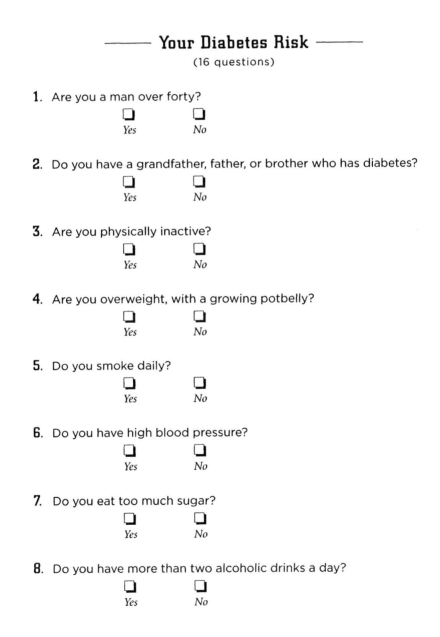

——— **Your Diabetes Risk** ———

(16 questions)

1. Are you a man over forty?

    ❏ Yes   ❏ No

2. Do you have a grandfather, father, or brother who has diabetes?

    ❏ Yes   ❏ No

3. Are you physically inactive?

    ❏ Yes   ❏ No

4. Are you overweight, with a growing potbelly?

    ❏ Yes   ❏ No

5. Do you smoke daily?

    ❏ Yes   ❏ No

6. Do you have high blood pressure?

    ❏ Yes   ❏ No

7. Do you eat too much sugar?

    ❏ Yes   ❏ No

8. Do you have more than two alcoholic drinks a day?

    ❏ Yes   ❏ No

9. Do you have high cholesterol?

☐   ☐
Yes   *No*

10. Are you stressed out a lot?

☐   ☐
Yes   *No*

11. Do you have to urinate too frequently, especially at night after going to sleep?

☐   ☐
Yes   *No*

12. Do you think you feel constantly thirsty?

☐   ☐
Yes   *No*

13. Do you feel extreme hunger, as if you'll fall over if you don't eat something right away?

☐   ☐
Yes   *No*

14. Have you been recently losing weight without any explanation?

☐   ☐
Yes   *No*

15. Do you have episodes of blurry vision?

☐   ☐
Yes   *No*

16. Are you African American, Asian American, Hispanic, Native American, or a Pacific Islander?

☐   ☐
Yes   *No*

See your risk for diabetes by totaling the number of Yes answers.

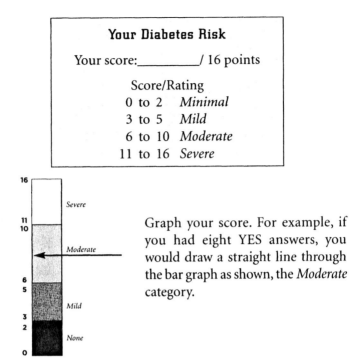

Your Diabetes Risk

Your score:_____/ 16 points

Score/Rating
0 to 2   *Minimal*
3 to 5   *Mild*
6 to 10   *Moderate*
11 to 16   *Severe*

Graph your score. For example, if you had eight YES answers, you would draw a straight line through the bar graph as shown, the *Moderate* category.

Knowing where you are on the risk spectrum will help you decide how intensely you should follow these recommendations. If you're in the Severe range, with a score of 11 to 16, you should pay close attention to all the components of the program.

Of course, should you have any reason to suspect that you may have diabetes, consult with your health-care practitioner and get yourself tested.

UNDERSTAND THE KEY ISSUES

When You Have Diabetes, Your Body Ignores Your Insulin

Normally, when you eat sugar, it enters the bloodstream looking for a home. The hormone insulin is then released from the pancreas.

Insulin opens the doors for sugar, and allows it to enter cells. Once inside cells, the sugar can be used as the basic fuel for energy. This is true for every cell of the body. So far, there is no great antagonism between insulin and T.

The problem: a diabetic lockout.

In diabetes, your insulin doesn't open the doors so well. Thinking that you need help, the pancreas pours out huge quantities of more ineffective, weak insulin.

This is known as insulin resistance.

Your body doesn't use this weak insulin to break down glucose. It's as if insulin shows up for work but goes on strike and just walks the picket line. As a result, unprocessed sugar remains floating in the bloodstream, can't cross the cell line, and is locked out.

Insulin resistance means your body *resists* the effects of insulin, which doesn't open cell doors to allow sugar to go in.

This excess insulin smashes testosterone.

This excess, useless insulin affects testosterone negatively on multiple levels. This includes telling the brain to cut back on sending signals to the testes to make T.

One of the major complications of diabetes is peripheral-artery disease. This means there are blockages in the blood vessels that go to the legs. This includes the feeder pipes to the testes, too.

High levels of insulin even increase the amount of the chaperone protein of testosterone called SHBG (sex-hormone binding globulin). This chaperone molecule escorts, binds to, and jealously guards about half the T in the bloodstream, preventing it from doing its thing, from acting on tissues.

This takes even more testosterone out of active duty.

Diabetes opposes testosterone.

The Consequences of Insulin Resistance

One of the effects of diabetes is that insulin antagonizes T. They work at cross-purposes. Insulin dampens the production, distribution, and effects of testosterone.

To varying degrees, insulin resistance is occurring in about *50 million* North American men who are

- Diabetic
- Prediabetic
- Obese
- Overweight

Excess insulin is a major setback for testosterone.

Insulin and Sex Hormones

THE REMARKABLE LINK between insulin and sex hormones applies to women, also. This startling discovery has only recently been appreciated.

Polycystic ovarian syndrome is one type of fertility problem in women. There is a cluster of symptoms—including estrogen imbalance, cysts on the ovaries, excess facial hair, menstrual irregularity, and obesity. It turns out that the underlying cause is excess insulin.

So doctors are now treating infertility in women by using medicine that we would only give to diabetic clients. This is in women *who do not have* diabetes.

When women are prescribed Metformin, a diabetes medication, it goes after the excess insulin, and the symptom cluster improves. Estrogen rebalances, the ovarian cysts diminish, facial hair reduces, menstrual periods regularize, and the women lose weight. Then they have a much better chance of getting pregnant and completing the pregnancy to deliver a healthy baby.

This is the female side of the link between sex hormones and insulin levels.

As for the male connection: Doctors are now recommending that a diabetic man who has excessive fatigue, loss of interest in sex, or erection problems, must *directly* and *specifically* manage his testosterone needs.

The Infamous Potbelly

Call it love handles, the midsection paunch, flab, blubber, potbelly, beer belly, the midlife spread—abdominal fat is toxic. It is chemically malicious, more metabolically active than fat elsewhere in the body, and churns out disagreeable substances. This includes taking testosterone out of the bloodstream and converting it into the enemy hormone, estrogen. (See the Obesity chapter for a fuller explanation.)

A potbelly sets men up for a huge number of conditions. So far, doctors have called this cluster of problems *syndrome X*, or the metabolic syndrome.

About *30 million men* in North America have this syndrome. This is the lead-up to many complications, including heart attacks and diabetes.

Doctors keep seeing midlife men with a particular cluster of conditions. At first, it seemed these were isolated symptoms. So the mystery name, syndrome X, was coined. But it turns out that these conditions are caused by excess insulin.

The conditions include:

- Abdominal obesity
- High sugar, often leading to diabetes
- High blood pressure
- A tendency to develop blood clots

- Cholesterol imbalance: High LDL, low HDL
- High triglyceride fats
- Blood-vessel blockages everywhere
- Heart disease and heart attacks
- High chance of sudden cardiac death

Is declining T the cause of it all?

Research is under way, but it seems that declining testosterone levels may be the *lead cause* of syndrome X. Reduced T can explain the development of each condition in the cluster, including insulin resistance. Previously, insulin resistance had been thought to be the prime cause.

Diminishing T is already known to accelerate the development of diabetes in middle-aged men.

Syndrome X may eventually be known as testosterone deficiency syndrome. *Testosterone opposes diabetes.*

IF YOU ALREADY HAVE DIABETES, CONTROL IT

"Hey, doc, since I went off the T-program, my sugar has gone up a lot."

Increasing your T-impact helps reduce the sugar levels in your blood. The beneficial effect of T on diabetes includes:

- More effective insulin
- More insulin
- Better distributed insulin
- Insulin that is listened to

Because the insulin is more effective, it reduces your sugar levels. In turn, this helps to control and prevent syndrome X and diabetes.

Men who already have diabetes should know that building testosterone helps treat their diabetes. Building T helps to

- Control sugar
- Reduce the amount of medication they are taking
- Prevent the need for more medication
- Avoid having to start insulin injections because of tablet failure
- Reduce the number of organ complications of diabetes

Testosterone is antidiabetic: T is a strike-breaker. It forces insulin off its picket line and back to work, which lets glucose enter the cells.

T makes your body listen to your own insulin, sensitizing your body to it. As a result, T reverses insulin resistance, which is the master defect in diabetes.

T also works at the level of a cell's genes, ordering more sugar-handling infrastructure to be created. When insulin arrives, it finds itself in welcome territory, and opens the doors for glucose to enter the cell.

This mechanism of action is similar to that of new-generation diabetes medications such as Avandia and Actos.

Why Get Tested Annually?

TESTING YOURSELF EVERY year will alert you to problems early. This way, there is no lost time between diagnosis and management, between the alert and the remedy.

For example, on average, a man will have already had diabetes for *five years* before he is diagnosed. This means five years of uncontrolled damage to internal organs.

This is a tragedy that can be easily averted with annual tests.

IF YOU DON'T ALREADY HAVE DIABETES, AVOID DEVELOPING IT

This is a profoundly hopeful statement that can help 30 million North American men.

THERMOGENESIS, OR HEAT PRODUCTION:
This is another way T helps prevent diabetes. T stimulates the body to burn both fat and sugar.

By increasing your testosterone, you can avoid developing the cluster of symptoms known as syndrome X and diabetes. You can avoid developing insulin resistance, obesity, heart complications, high fats, and clotting tendencies.

To help prevent the onset of these conditions, it is important to discover hints of any problems early. You can do this with the following tests, in particular by doing a tremendously important test known as the hemoglobin A1c.

MONITOR YOUR DIABETES POTENTIAL
BY GETTING SCREENING TESTS ANNUALLY

Every man over forty should get these tests once a year.

To be fully aware of your potential for syndrome X, diabetes, and dampened T, measure your

- Fasting glucose
- Hemoglobin A1c
- Fasting insulin
- Urine glucose (glucosuria)
- Urine protein (microalbuminuria)
- Triglycerides

Fasting Glucose

This is the classic test for sugar diabetes. It must be done fasting, which means you cannot have any food overnight for eight to twelve hours before this test. This standardization ensures that sugars from your meals don't interfere with the result.

The problem is that this test picks up on problems *late*. The fasting glucose tends to reveal problems only after a person is fully diabetic.

We need tests that pick up diabetic potential much *earlier*.

100 mg/dl (milligrams/deciliter) or more means that a sugar problem has started, that you are prediabetic.

126 mg/dl or more means that you have diabetes.

Hemoglobin A1c

It will take five more years for doctors to understand that they should be offering this test as an annual screening. Ask for it to be done every year. This is the best test to pick up *prediabetes.*

This is a brilliant test, a measurement of your sugar over the past three months.

It is a much more powerful and sensitive indicator than doing either a fasting glucose or an on-the-spot finger-prick test. It will pick up problems much earlier than these other standard tests.

The earlier you know of any sugar control problems, the earlier you will be able to counteract them.

So far, this is the best screening test we have, and should be done by all men over forty once a year.

Medical laboratories still have to get their act together on this test. Normal test values change from one state to another, even from one part of the same city to another. The problem is bureaucratic.

This lack of standardization is preventing the official endorsement of this test as an official screen. For the time being, try to have your yearly tests at the same laboratory to prevent lab-to-lab discrepancies from skewing your scores.

Note: You can't cheat on this test. Someone who dreads the results may skip a meal or take extra medication so that his on-the-spot sugar will look good on a finger-prick test, which is known as a random glucose measurement. But there is no way you can fudge a three-month reading.

Above 6 percent means that a sugar problem has *just* started, that you
are prediabetic.
Above 7 percent means that a sugar problem has fully developed, that
you are diabetic.

What is the extra information this test provides?
This test is an accurate measure of the sugar in your bloodstream over the past three months. It firmly shows if you have any hint of diabetes or not—if you are nondiabetic, prediabetic, or diabetic. It also tells us if you are en route to developing syndrome X.

This is also the test that doctors use to determine if clients will develop the complications of diabetes. These include heart disease, kidney damage, eye damage, nerve damage, foot sores, amputations, and erectile dysfunction.

For example, in the same way that you can have a candied apple—an apple that was dipped in sugar syrup and is now coated over with a glucose layer—diabetes can create candied organs. And sugarcoated organs, tissues, cells, and arteries don't function properly.

In particular, with the hemoglobin A1c test you can measure the risk for a special complication—diminished nerve and blood supply to the testes. This is part of a group of disorders known as peripheral vascular disease, which has a direct impact on your T-status.

For Doctors Only—A Plea to Physician Colleagues

AS YOU KNOW, the hemoglobin A1c, the glycosylated hemoglobin, measures the cumulative effect of postprandial glucose spikes. It is the integration of area-under-the-curve graphs. It picks up derangements in sugar indices *much earlier* than fasting or random glucose measurements. It is also far more convenient than the oral glucose tolerance test.

We aspire to practice preventive medicine, and it is now time to act. Don't let bureaucracy get in the way. Please convene, standardize the reference range values, and let's begin regular, annual screening in North America for prediabetes, diabetes, and syndrome X.

Any less than this, and we are collectively doing a great disservice to the clients we serve. Our continued silence and inaction are violating our Hippocratic oath, *Primum non nocere*—Above all else, do no harm.

Fasting Insulin

Above 15 µU/ml (microUnits/milliliter) means that there is extra insulin in the bloodstream, a sign of insulin resistance and the beginning of syndrome X.

Note that this is a measurement of "fasting free insulin."

Track insulin resistance by tracking insulin.

One of the earliest changes in syndrome X is the secretion of excessive amounts of weak, ineffective, and ignored insulin. We can measure these insulin levels directly. Yet, doctors don't do this. Why?

- Men may not go to doctors to get the tests.
- Doctors may have forgotten that this test is available and that it can be done easily.
- Doctors may not know the significance of the results, how to interpret them, or what to do afterward.
- Insurance companies and third-party payers may not pay for the test.
- Doctors may be busy chasing the individual components of syndrome X—obesity, high sugar, high cholesterol, high triglycerides, high blood pressure, and so on—and not realize that syndrome X is a package deal.
- Doctors may not have woken up to the fact that insulin resistance is one of the prime movers of syndrome X.
- Doctors may not be aggressive enough, and not practice *preventive* medicine.
- Or, doctors may simply not be putting all this information to use for the benefit of their clients.

Whatever the reason(s) for not doing this test, an elevated fasting insulin is an important and powerful early marker of many unhealthy metabolic changes to come.

Urine Glucose (Glucosuria)

Your urine should be clear, with no sugar being spilled by the kidneys.

Doctors are often alerted to a client's unrecognized diabetes by the persistent presence of significant amounts of sugar in the urine. The urine test may have been done incidentally, perhaps as part of an insurance physical examination.

We may find sugar—glucose—spilling into the urine long before we see huge increases in the blood sugar measurements.

Basically, the kidneys are overwhelmed by the amount of sugar coming their way, unable to reabsorb it all—which is what they're supposed to do—and start leaking it out into the urine.

Protein in the Urine (Microalbuminuria)

Again, your urine should be clear, with no protein being spilled by the kidneys.

We often find a specific type of protein, what doctors call microalbumin, spilling into the urine.

The spilling of protein into the urine can be a complication of diabetes, high blood pressure, kidney disease, or all three conditions. Doctors can be alerted to a client's unrecognized condition by the persistent presence of significant amounts of protein in the urine. Again, this test may have been done incidentally, perhaps as part of an annual physical.

This is a good, inexpensive screening test, an early sign of more trouble to come.

Triglycerides

Triglycerides are blood fats—lipids—the poor cousin of cholesterol. They hardly get the attention that cholesterol does, but they are also an important component of plaque buildup, blood vessel blockages, and atherosclerosis.

Diabetic clients often have significantly elevated triglyceride levels as part of their chemical profile. We are often alerted to impending diabetes or syndrome X when we see clients with unexpectedly high triglyceride levels.

> More than 150 mg/dl (milligrams/deciliter) means that this fat is elevated, and may be a sign of insulin resistance, and the beginning of syndrome X.

REDUCE YOUR CHANCES OF DEVELOPING SYNDROME X AND DIABETES

"But, doc, how can I have my coffee without sugar?"

You can and you should. This recommendation kicks in at age forty, and stays in effect for life.

Now, if it's the occasional treat—somebody's birthday, Super Bowl Sunday, a holiday party, whatever—fine, you get a sugar pass. But these should be several days apart. Do not continue to have sugar daily.

North American men could avoid so much disease, so many conditions, if they severely limited the amount of sugar they eat. In 1900, we ate fifteen pounds of sugar per person every year. Now it's ten times that—about 150 pounds of sugar per person per year. This is obscene and damaging. It's more than unhealthy—it's slow, self-administered poison.

See the Diet chapter for a full discussion.

Learn about the Glycemic Index

Foods are now rated according to their sugar-power—how much sugar they contain, and how long the sugar-high will last once the food has been eaten. This is known as the glycemic index. So far, more than four thousand foods have been evaluated and assigned a glycemic index.

Here are several important lists drawn from our knowledge of the glycemic index—foods with obvious sugars and hidden sugars.

Avoid high-glycemic-index foods that contain *obvious* sugars (see page 62).

Generally, these foods—especially the snack and convenience foods—provide empty, hollow calories with little nutritional benefit.

Also avoid high-glycemic-index foods that contain *hidden* sugars (see page 63).

People often don't realize that these simple carbohydrates are also sugar once they are broken down and digested. These foods should not be a regular part of your diet.

Unfortunately, people of many cultures are accustomed to eating rice or bread daily, even twice a day. It may be hard to break from tradition, but it is vital to your health that you do so.

In total, do not eat any of these secretly sugar-loaded foods more than twice a week. Instead, substitute whole-grain products for those made with white flour, sweet potatoes for white potatoes, and brown rice for white rice—permanently.

To reduce your potential for developing syndrome X and Diabetes, follow these chapters closely:

- Chapter 2 Sleep
- Chapter 4 Exercise
- Chapter 6 Diet
- Chapter 10 Supplements
- Chapter 13 Stress Levels
- Chapter 14 Therapeutic Self-Massage

10

Supplements

SUPPLEMENTS PLAY AN important role in your nutrition. Choosing the right supplements can be crucial to your overall health, and can thus maximize T.

All men can benefit by understanding the choices in this chapter, but especially those who had high scores in the Medical Background, Habits and Lifestyle, and Diet questionnaires.

"If I'm going to take all these supplements, spend good money on them, can't I eat and drink whatever I want?"

No. It is not clear if men are genetically predisposed to search for loopholes, but they do.

Supplements, like prescription medications, are not a substitute for healthy eating habits and lifestyle.

Also, don't think that if you follow the advice in one chapter, that this buys you the freedom not to follow the advice in another chapter.

Supplements should be used in combination with the other T-enhancing approaches in this book. Supplements alone are not enough.

WHY SUPPLEMENTS ARE IMPORTANT

HEALTH-CARE PRACTITIONERS value health supplements because we have some understanding of the incredible complexity, fragility, and beauty of the inside workings of the human body.

If you were to peer into the inner workings of your own cells, you would be astounded at the number of biochemical reactions and processes going on all the time. In fact, it would be difficult to wrap your head around the staggering numbers involved, the efficiency, and the interrelated nature of human biology.

For example, a healthy man produces 11 billion molecules of testosterone every second—that's 11,000,000,000 per second.

Eleven billion.

It's astonishing.

And the body would not devote resources to a production schedule like that unless it thought it was extremely important.

The body would only produce a substance in such quantities if it knew there was a hungry internal market, a devoted following, innumerable applications, and that the product was constantly needed.

With so many biochemical reactions going on, many can go bad.

On one level, that's actually what aging is. There are mistakes in production cycles, delays in shipments, wasted resources, raw materials delivered to the wrong addresses, lost parcels, busy signals, offline systems, network crashes, and ignored orders. Eventually, the body is overwhelmed. It ages. There is a slow but steady general shutdown.

Start taking health supplements early in your life, earlier than you think you need to. Supplements will help you maintain good health, not merely mend ill health.

Key Points

- Supplements boost our natural defenses against the outside world.
- Supplements protect the body against self-attack.
- Supplements neutralize the silent damage perpetrated by microscopic toxins.
- Certain supplements enhance testosterone production and effects.
- Certain supplements enhance intelligent deployment of testosterone.
- Supplements help protect us against cancer, the number one killer in North America.

Helping to Prevent Cancer

CHRONIC SMOKING IS toxic to the cells that produce testosterone, leaving microscopic damage. This leads to lower sperm counts, weaker sperm, and more malformed sperm.

But, along with aging, cancer is also one of the results of biochemical derangements. Our modern lifestyle and poor diets can cause, accelerate, and amplify these errors.

Supplements can help to counteract these ill effects.

WHAT TO DO

- Take enteric coated aspirin (EC ASA).
- Take a high-quality multivitamin.
- Decide which supplements you should take based on your specific needs.
- Increase or decrease the number of supplements that you take according to your own needs and response.

TAKE ENTERIC COATED ASPIRIN (EC ASA)

In your bloodstream right now, there are approximately 1 billion platelets floating around. These are like tiny pieces of adhesive tape, looking for any crack, any weakening, or any rip in the pipes. If there is a slight nick or cut anywhere in the arteries, it's the platelets that clump and clot together to stop the bleeding.

With a billion microscopic pieces of sticky tape floating around in the blood, this plugging up happens all the time on every internal microscopic tear. Unfortunately, this repair sometimes gets carried away and can lead to blocked arteries.

Aspirin (ASA) is the most cost-effective supplement in the modern world. It's cheap, easily available, generic, and available over the counter.

Aspirin thins the blood and protects against heart disease and blood vessel blockages. Taking a small dosage regularly largely retards this clotting. Basically, aspirin helps to keep the blood running on time. It reduces your chance of having a heart attack by *30 percent.*

Take 325 mg of EC ASA once per day.

This recommendation is for *most* men over forty. However, this is not for everyone, as explained below.

Aspirin Resistance

Most doctors recommend baby aspirin, the 81 mg dosage. We have found that this is too little—too weak a dose to achieve optimal blood thinning.

About 25 to 40 percent of men are resistant to this "baby" dose of aspirin. That means millions of men will not be getting the blood-thinning benefit they think they're getting.

Men with high cholesterol levels are often the ones who are resistant to aspirin, and the ones who need the higher dose, 325 mg.

Can You Tolerate Aspirin?

EC means enteric coated, having a special coating on the aspirin tablet that makes it easier to digest.

Aspirin can be tough on the stomach, and some men will experience acid, burning, excess gas, even ulcers. If you have a sensitive stomach or a history of bleeding ulcers, you may not be able to tolerate the higher dose, the "baby" dose, or even *any* dose of aspirin. If you have aspirin-related problems, speak to your health-care practitioner to discuss the best approach for you.

Benefit from the Anti-Inflammatory Action of Aspirin

When the body goes to war against a disease or against an outside invading organism, the process is called inflammation. The area under attack becomes red, swollen, tender, painful, and angry.

Sometimes this process initiates damage leading to cancer. The higher dose of aspirin works against inflammation, as an anti-inflammatory. It has protective effects against a number of cancers, including cancer of the prostate gland.

TAKE A HIGH-QUALITY MULTIVITAMIN

Capitalize on the known and emerging benefits of a daily vitamin.

Few of us regularly get all the various vitamins and minerals that we should, what's known as the Daily Values (DV). Yet with the explosion of medical knowledge, we are learning more and more of the benefits of general multivitamins.

Whether we wish to maintain blood cells, keep our oxygen-carrying capacity high, keep the electricity flowing in our nerves efficiently, or help an unnamed number of essential biochemical reactions in the body—a good multivitamin will support all these processes.

Buy Vitamins from Reputable Outlets, Made by Respected Manufacturers

When purchasing supplements, don't fall for hyped advertising and lofty claims that sound too good to be true—they're not. People who purchase vitamins from roving salespeople, private labels, some Internet sites, and some herbal stores may not always get what they pay for.

I have had many clients who have paid for tablets that have no active ingredients at all, or which have doses much lower than claimed. Only purchase vitamin supplements from established outlets.

What a Multivitamin Supplement Should Contain

There may be slight variations in the contents of various multivitamins and the dosages' various components. For example, contents can vary among different brands, manufacturers, and formulations.

The contents listed here are the backbone of a high-quality product.
You can find out more about multivitamins by researching such Web sites
as www.consumerlab.com.

A high-quality multivitamin should contain:

- Vitamin A
- Vitamin C
- Vitamin D
- Vitamin E
- Vitamin B_1 (thiamine)
- Vitamin B_2 (riboflavin)
- Vitamin B_3 (niacin)
- Vitamin B_5 (pantothenic acid)
- Vitamin B_6 (pyridoxine)
- Vitamin B_9 (folic acid)
- Biotin (a B vitamin formerly known as vitamin H)
- Vitamin B_{12} (cobalamin)

FOLIC ACID SUPPLEMENTS help to reduce homocysteine, a cardiac risk factor.
See the chapter on Heart Trouble.

And the minerals:

- Calcium
- Chloride
- Chromium
- Copper
- Iodine
- Iron
- Magnesium
- Manganese
- Molybdenum
- Nickel
- Phosphorus
- Selenium
- Silicon
- Vanadium
- Zinc

Take your high quality, all-purpose multivitamin once per day.

DECIDE WHICH SUPPLEMENTS YOU SHOULD TAKE
BASED ON YOUR SPECIFIC NEEDS

Take these supplements *in addition* to aspirin and a multivitamin, which are recommended for all men over 40:

- Zinc
- Calcium
- Vitamin C
- Selenium
- Vitamin D
- Fish oil
- Vitamin E
- Vitamin B complex 100
- Choose *either*, but not both: (a) nettle root extract; *or* (b) indole-3-carbinol (I3C).

"Isn't this a lot of supplements?"

Yes.

Typically, clients will start supplements, and then increase or decrease the number they take based on their response and needs.

As you progress through the T-enhancing program, you will be able to cut back on the number of supplements.

INCREASE OR DECREASE THE NUMBER OF SUPPLEMENTS THAT YOU
USE ACCORDING TO YOUR OWN NEEDS AND RESPONSE

Some men will use the basic suggestions: Aspirin, the multivitamin, with the addition of, say, zinc and calcium. Other men will find that they benefit from taking more of these recommended supplements, and some even take all nine per day.

This choice needs to be tailored to your individual requirements, as well as how you respond to the various supplements.

Not duplication:

Even though your multivitamin may contain some of the other supplements mentioned here, this is not duplication. The value of the multivitamin is that it has a little bit of everything, but in small doses.

For example, I later recommend 100 mg of vitamin B₁, as part of a B complex supplement. A general multivitamin might typically contain only 2.25 mg of vitamin B₁, about 2 percent of the full dosage.

Zinc

Zinc does not get much attention but it should.

The North American diet and lifestyle seem to lead to partial zinc deficiencies.

Alcohol, physical stress, and aging itself all reduce the body's zinc supply. In addition, processed, packaged foods do not contain any zinc.

Zinc is an essential trace mineral element, like iron. It is surprisingly important for optimal testosterone production and release, and even fertility. Zinc participates in at least five hundred different biochemical reactions in the body, and therefore has widespread effects.

The Many Functions of Zinc

There is a chemical thief in the abdominal fat of men, the enzyme aromatase. This working molecule steals circulating testosterone out of the blood and turns it into the female hormone estrogen. Zinc lowers the amount of this enzyme, and the efficiency of the theft. This is how zinc helps to keep more T circulating freely in the bloodstream.

Ultimately, the orders placed in real time for increased or decreased testosterone come from the brain. Specifically, the master hormone controller is the pituitary gland, which is about the size of a pea, and sits just behind the eyes. Zinc helps to keep signals going from the pituitary gland to the testes efficient and strong.

With billions of T molecules being produced each second, it is vital that the DNA genetic blueprint from which testosterone is copied stays clean, free from breaks and spelling mistakes. Zinc helps to keep this high output printing press in working order by repairing damage to the template of the genetic material.

Finally, by its enhancing effect on T and the local environment inside the testes, zinc helps to increase the sperm count, and makes sperm more energetic. Doctors call this enhanced motility, or movement. In essence, zinc helps to make sperm into better long-distance swimmers.

Take 50 mg of zinc once per day.

Zinc is especially recommended for men who drink regularly, lead very busy lives, are obese, or are having problems with fertility.

Calcium

Your bones are alive.

There are 206 bones in the body, and they are not static but alive. Bones constantly rebuild or slowly dissolve away from the inside, depending on what they experience. Bones are strongest by age thirty, and start to slowly weaken after that. That's exactly the age when testosterone itself starts to decline.

By taking adequate amounts of calcium, you relieve testosterone from its bone-repairing duty.

T is then freer to work elsewhere.

What Is Osteoporosis?

Literally, this means porous bones. An *osteoporotic* skeleton is like imitation bone, a calcium veneer with hollowing insides and unrepaired holes— like termites in the woodwork. Insufficient calcium can lead to this condition.

Virtually all the recommendations regarding calcium, counseling about bone health, and educational campaigns are directed toward women. Unbelievably, doctors have simply *forgotten* that men have bones, too.

Generally, doctors do not advise men to monitor their calcium intake, and men go on to silently develop osteoporosis. This bone loss can lead to generalized bone and joint pain, as well as fractures of specific locations such as the hips, spine, and wrists.

This loss of calcium from bone happens daily, little by little, in bits and pieces, all the time. About *20 million men* in North America are at risk for developing osteoporosis—in addition to the 5 million men who have osteoporosis right now.

This calcium loss is accelerated by caffeine, nicotine, emotional stress, lack of physical exercise, lack of sun exposure—and diminishing testosterone.

Testosterone builds bone, helps to absorb calcium in the diet, and helps to distribute calcium where it's needed, fortifying the skeleton.

If you let your bones weaken by not having enough calcium, the testosterone molecules are directed to and get used up in building bone. Then there is less T available to work elsewhere in the body.

Taking enough calcium frees T from bone duty. This is what we mean by the statement, *Certain supplements enhance intelligent deployment of testosterone.*

With due respect to physician colleagues:

Trying to pinpoint a testosterone deficiency, a famous medical questionnaire for men asks, *Have you lost height?* This is an incredible question to ask. Why do doctors wait until men shrivel and shrink to help them?

> Translated, what the questionnaire is asking is:
> Are the bones in your back weak enough to have collapsed in
> on themselves? Are the bones in your spine turning to jelly? Have
> you had a mudslide in your vertebrae yet, to the point where
> you've lost two inches of your adult height?
> Surely this is too late. Surely doctors can intervene earlier, help
> men keep their bones strong, and preserve their height. This will also
> keep testosterone intelligently deployed, and not lost in the bone war.
> Men deserve to stand tall.

Under age 50, take 1000 mg of calcium once per day.
Over age 50, take 1,500 mg of calcium once per day.

This supplement is recommended especially for men who may not get adequate calcium in their diet, for example, who have less than the equivalent of four glasses of 2% milk per day, as well as for men who have had excess caffeine, nicotine, or alcohol in their lives.

Vitamin C

Vitamin C has many applications.

This vitamin participates in several hundred biochemical reactions, and more are being discovered and cataloged regularly. These include helping the body cleanse itself of cholesterol that sticks to the walls of arteries, strengthening bones, promoting wound healing, helping to clear alcohol faster, softening allergies, protecting against various cancers, and tolerating cancer chemotherapy better.

Most important to our discussion, vitamin C helps to reduce and neutralize one of T's major opponents, the stress hormone cortisol. It helps to keep the shifting balance between T and cortisol in favor of T.

In North America, vitamin C is a particularly important natural antidote to the chemical after-effects of our chronically stressed lives.

Under age 50, take 500 mg of vitamin C once per day.
Over age 50, take 1,000 mg of vitamin C once per day.

This supplement is recommended especially for men who feel they are under perpetual physical and emotional stress.

This is a higher dose than is found in most multivitamins, which usually contain around *90 mg* of vitamin C. The lower *90 mg* dose is enough to prevent scurvy, a disease that first came to attention in 1753 in the British

Navy. Sailors on long sea voyages, who had no access to fresh fruits, developed this condition. (The sailors' teeth fell out; they also had stiff joints, bleeding under the skin, and weak blood.) That's how old our thinking is on the recommended dose of vitamin C.

It's time for an update and an increase in the recommended dose. This higher dose promotes good health, and reflects current science.

Many men report that they start feeling relief from both psychological and physical stress as early as seven to ten days after beginning the 500 mg dose.

Selenium

Like iron and zinc, selenium is a trace metal element that participates in several biochemical reactions.

Selenium has direct effects on testosterone and fertility. Selenium and the molecular complexes it forms help in the testosterone manufacturing process known as the biosynthesis pathway. It is also essential for the maturation of anatomically normal and vibrant sperm. Sperm produced in a low-selenium environment have motility problems. They don't move properly, as they have malformed tails and other structural defects.

Selenium also helps to detoxify the body. This mineral is one of the chief structural elements in a group of detoxifying enzymes, particularly those known as the glutathione peroxidases. This group of enzymes functions, as the body's own cleanup team for chemical spills. Environmental toxins, such as gasoline exhaust, pesticides, and hormone disruptors—which are mostly estrogens—are partly neutralized through this team of molecules.

Take 200 micrograms of selenium once per day.

This supplement is recommended especially for men who are regularly exposed to industrial chemicals, who have eaten "too much" meat in their lives, who smoke, and are having fertility problems.

Vitamin D

It is estimated that 30 percent of North American men are deficient in vitamin D.

Natural vitamin D is made in the skin, set off by 15-minute bursts of sunlight. While the dangers of overexposure to sunlight are very real, it is also true that we are not getting enough ray-time. Winter, sunblock, indoor shopping malls, underground parking, and subways all contribute to this deficiency.

Though vitamin D has myriad effects, it makes two main contributions to T status:

Vitamin D Works with Calcium to Build Bone

Vitamin D assists calcium. It helps the bloodstream to absorb calcium from the intestine, to distribute calcium to the inner areas of bone, and to set—or mineralize—calcium into proper, solid bone structure.

With these contributions, vitamin D helps to relieve testosterone from servicing bone. Testosterone is then freed up to exert its hormonal action elsewhere.

Vitamin D Helps Convert T's Opponent, Estrogen, into a Weaker Form

Estrogen is actually a group of hormones, almost thirty different identified compounds. It is usually divided into three components: estrone (estrogen 1), estradiol (estrogen 2), and estriol (estrogen 3). These have different strengths, exist in a fluctuating balance, and can convert into each other.

In men, vitamin D helps to soften estrogenic effects. It converts the stronger estrogens into the weaker form, estriol.

Vitamin D helps T to continue to rule.

Under age 50, take 400 IU (International Units) of vitamin D per day.
Over age 50, take 800 IU (International Units) of vitamin D per day.

Multivitamins generally contain 400 IU of vitamin D, so the multivitamin alone will suffice if you are under fifty. To get 800 IU of vitamin D will require a supplement.

Vitamin D is especially recommended for men who have too many aches and pains, who have known bone problems, and who live in parts of the country with long winters and reduced sun exposure.

Fish Oils

Omega-3 and omega-6 fatty acid fish oils are special. There is an ever-expanding inventory of their widespread health benefits. These include:

- Promoting good blood circulation
- Lowering LDL cholesterol
- Raising HDL cholesterol
- Preventing heart attacks
- Thinning blood to prevent clots
- Lowering blood pressure
- Keeping the heart beat rhythm regular
- Fighting off inflammation
- Fighting off immune self-attack
- Promoting smooth joint movement

- Stabilizing cell membranes
- Helping you to tolerate stress better
- Elevating your mood

Men who take fish oil supplements have:

- Fewer heart attacks
- Smaller heart attacks
- Less damaging heart attacks
- Better survival after heart attacks

Two of these oils are essential for testosterone manufacture.

Omega-3 and omega-6 are known as EFAs, essential fatty acids. They are essential because the body cannot make them on its own. These fatty oils must be obtained from the diet.

Preparations and dosages will vary, but cold-pressed fish oil capsules should contain:

- Omega 3 oils
  EPA (eicosapentaenoic acid)
  DHA (docosahexaenoic acid)
  ALA (alpha-linolenic acid)
- Omega 6 oils
  LA (linoleic acid)
  GLA (gamma-linolenic acid)

The terminology can get complex, but these fatty acids are integral parts of the testosterone biosynthesis pathway. You just need to remember the number: omega-3 and omega-6.

Under age 50, take one capsule of omega-3/omega-6 cold-pressed fish oils, once per day.
Over age 50, take two capsules of omega-3/omega-6 cold-pressed fish oils, once per day.

There are enough combination formulations available—with both omega-3 and omega 6 oils—that you should be able to find all these in a single capsule.

If only separate preparations are available at your pharmacy, take one capsule of omega-3 oils and one of omega-6.

Fish oils are recommended especially for men who have or are at risk for developing heart problems: that includes all men with high blood pressure, obesity, and excess stress.

> WARNING: if you have a bleeding tendency, diabetes, or an aspirin allergy, speak with your health-care practitioner to see if you can tolerate fish oil supplements, or if the dosage needs to be adjusted.

Vitamin E

Vitamin E helps to clear the body of incidental products of its own biochemical reactions.

Just as factories produce industrial waste, the body itself produces aggressive and toxic chemicals. Free radicals are toxic by-products of the body's own biochemical processes. These high-energy substances act as internal microscopic terrorists, damaging cells, promoting cancers, leading to inflammation, and immune self-attack.

Basically, free radicals rust—or oxidize—your insides.

Vitamin E is an antioxidant, in the anti-rust business. It helps to round up and neutralize these internal terrorists, preserving tissue integrity and keeping your cells and DNA intact.

Vitamin E and Insulin

Vitamin E helps insulin work efficiently to counteract high sugar levels. This is known as potentiation. This process helps keep insulin from interfering with and dampening the action of testosterone.

In a sense, vitamin E helps keep insulin off testosterone's back.

Under age 50, take 100 IU (International Units) of vitamin E once per day.
Over age 50, take 200 IU (International Units) of vitamin E once per day.

Vitamin E is especially recommended for men who are obese, and who have or are at risk for developing diabetes.

> SOME MEN ARE unable to tolerate vitamin E taken in conjunction with aspirin. If you have a bleeding tendency, speak to your health-care practitioner to decide what's best for you.
>
> Also, if you have this intolerance, do not take the usual recommended dose of 400 IU of vitamin E. With long-term use alongside aspirin, this dosage increases your risk for heart failure.

Vitamin B Complex 100

The B complex vitamins, considered all together, participate in more than 15,000 biological processes. It would literally take another book to itemize the details.

The positive effects include:

- Efficient blood cell production
- Smooth nerve conduction
- Preserving mental function
- Enhanced liver protection
- Efficient energy metabolism
- Proper digestion
- Better nutrient distribution
- Enhanced testosterone synthesis
- Having good hair, nails, skin, and vision

B complex 100 contains 100 mg of each important B vitamin, plus smaller amounts of other B vitamins. Typically, a supplement will offer:

- Vitamin B_1 (thiamine) 100 mg
- Vitamin B_2 (riboflavin) 100 mg
- Vitamin B_3 (niacin) 100 mg
- Vitamin B_5 (pantothenic acid) 100 mg
- Vitamin B_6 (pyridoxine) 100 micrograms
- Vitamin B_9 (folic acid) 400 micrograms
- Biotin 100 micrograms
- Vitamin B_{12} (cobalamin) 100 micrograms

A multivitamin will also contain the important B vitamins, but at a much lower dosage. For example, a typical multivitamin contains 2.25 mg of vitamin B_1 (thiamine).

Take a 100 mg B complex supplement once per day.

B complex supplements are especially recommended for men who feel they are benefiting from their multivitamin but would like to boost its effects. B complex vitamins are especially recommended if you have a stressful lifestyle.

Choose Either, but Not Both: (a) Nettle Root Extract, or (b) Indole-3-Carbinol (I3C)

These herbal supplements are derived from natural substances, but this is both a blessing and a curse.

It's a *blessing* because these supplements are not prescription medications, are relatively inexpensive, there is no patent protection, there are many preparations available, they are easily available, you can self-dose, and you can buy them over the Internet.

It's a *curse* because these supplements are not prescription medications, are relatively inexpensive, there is no patent protection, there are many preparations available, they are easily available, you can self-dose, and you can buy them over the Internet.

What does that mean?

Unlike pharmaceutical medicines, these herbals are natural substances that cannot be patented—so there is less money to be made from them. While that may keep the unit cost down, brand-name pharmaceutical and nutraceutical companies are less interested in bringing them to market. As a result, there is *no* FDA regulation regarding research, product quality, standardization of dosing, safety, or side effects. If it's an herbal remedy, it does not even have to contain what the bottle label says it contains. No regulatory body checks even that.

Often, convincingly marketed bottles of these herbal products turn out to contain little or no active ingredients.

It is important to obtain these herbal supplements from reliable outlets, preferably through a medical pharmacy.

Nettle Root Extract

Nettle Root extract is recommended only *for men who have high-end, Severe scores in most of the questionnaire subsections, and also for those men who feel that the other supplements have not helped enough.*

There are a number of names for this particular plant: stinging nettle root, *Urtica radix*, and *Urtica dioica radix*. It's important to purchase extract that is made from the root, not from the stem, hairs, leaves, or seeds. It is the root extract that has the medicinal effect.

About half the testosterone floating in the blood is actually being held hostage, under guard and adult supervision. This stranded T is tightly bound to a chaperone protein, and is unable to exert any biological effect.

This chaperone protein is called SHBG, sex-hormone binding globulin. The T that it holds hostage is called bound testosterone, and it is inactive, just there for the ride. It's as if your body wouldn't trust you with all your T floating around freely, ready to perform, ready to rev up cells anytime.

Nettle root extract rescues testosterone from the chaperone protein. In fact, the extract offers itself up in exchange, as a decoy, and takes the place of T as substitute hostage.

In this manner, more T is dislodged from the chaperone protein, floats freely in the bloodstream, and once again becomes biologically active—or bioavailable.

Indole-3-Carbinol (I3C)

Indole-3-carbinol (I3C) is recommended only *for* overweight *men who have high-end, Severe scores in most of the questionnaire subsections, and also for* overweight *men who feel that the other supplements have not helped enough.*

Indole-3-carbinol is a plant chemical—a phytochemical—found naturally in such vegetables as bok choy, broccoli, Brussels sprouts, cauliflower, cabbage, kale, radishes, turnips, and watercress. These are known as cruciferous vegetables.

I3C is a mild anti-estrogen.

It turns out that there are at least two mechanisms by which I3C opposes estrogen. First, it is a mild aromatase inhibitor. Aromatase is the thief enzyme found in a man's abdominal fat, which steals T and turns it into estrogen. I3C opposes this enzyme conversion.

This mechanism is also why I3C seems to be particularly beneficial to overweight and obese men. Men with excess abdominal fat have more of the aromatase enzyme, and I3C goes directly after this T-thief.

Second, I3C helps to downregulate estrogen by converting the strong form—estradiol—into weaker forms.

Together, these mechanisms diminish estrogen's impact, removing some of T's competition and thus leaving more of the field open for T.

A third benefit is that I3C helps slow, diminish, or protect against estrogen-sensitive cancers.

Doctors have started noticing the value of I3C in its anticancer effects. It is being researched in women for use as additional therapy for cancer of the cervix (the opening of uterus), and for estrogen-sensitive breast cancers. It also seems to have application in men for prostate cancer.

MAINLAND CHINESE MEN consume large amounts of broccoli, Brussels sprouts, cauliflower, and cabbage.

They also consume far less meat than Westerners. And the meat they do consume has not been exposed to environmental hormone disruptors, the xenoestrogens.

As a result, they have dramatically lower rates of prostate cancer.

Their prostate cancer rates go up hugely once they move to North America and adopt a Western diet and lifestyle.

Dosage

If you are near your ideal weight, use nettle root extract: Take 250 mg of nettle root extract twice per day.

If you are significantly overweight, use indole-3-carbinol (I3C):

If you are *less* than 50 pounds overweight, take 200 mg of I3C once per day.

If you are *more* than 50 pounds overweight, take 200 mg of I3C twice per day.

Note: It is advisable to use I3C in a *three-weeks-on/one-week-off* regimen. This schedule helps to reset the hormone balance and to give the body a break from this hormone manipulation. This is similar to how oral contraceptives, birth control pills, are prescribed for women. This program of three-weeks-on, one-week-off applies whether you are taking this supplement once or twice per day.

A Final Word about Herbal Supplements

IT IS OUR experience that each man will respond differently to these herbal extracts.

No doubt part of this has to do with each man's metabolism, but it also has to do with getting quality products from reliable manufacturers. There are individual differences in metabolisms, but even two bottles from the same manufacturer may have dramatically different quantities of active agents.

You may even have to try a couple of versions of the same supplement, from different manufacturers, to find a preferred supplier and get the true benefit of these herbal substances.

11

Genital and Urinary Systems

MEN SHOULD UNDERSTAND the points in this chapter, especially those who had high scores in the Sex, Medical Background, and Habits and Lifestyle questionnaires.

$$\boxed{\textbf{KEEP IT CLEAN}}$$

DURING INTERCOURSE, IT'S fine to enjoy yourself. But understand, when you have sex, there's an *intense backdraft,* a huge uptake of germs. You don't even realize this.

From where the testes sit, sex is an exchange of body fluids. Tens of millions of bacteria, viruses, and fungi—germs whose names no one can pronounce—change owners. This happens every time you have sex—even if it's with your regular partner, even with your partner of many years. It doesn't mean she's giving you dangerous bugs, just the "normal" ones. But you still take in millions.

From the testes' perspective, there are too many microbes floating around in sex. Your testes don't want to bring these germs into their home, their community, where immature sperm, the little ones, will grow up and from which they then go out to meet the world.

In your earlier days, did you have lots of partners? Did you have a lot of casual sex—sex just for fun? In your youth, did you receive oral sex from people whose names you can't even recall now? Yes? Whenever your penis touches or is touched by another person, even just that person's hand, you expose it to germs that can enter your urinary system and stay there. You probably picked up a lot of bugs through whatever kind of sex you have had. And, like so many men, you're carrying around bugs that you don't even know you have.

You may be all respectable now, with your settled life, having sown your wild oats earlier. But, hey, these bugs don't go away unless you treat them, and sometimes not even then.

If you don't destroy these germs, you muck up your genital neighborhood. You damage the T community, the sperm, and T-production infrastructure. I'm not just talking about men who learned they had a sexually transmitted disease. Millions of men are harboring germs in their groin.

You might benefit from cleansing your genital system.

Key Points

- Even sex with your regular partner exposes you to huge numbers of microbes.
- Repeatedly taking into your body of millions of bugs, even the usual ones, leads to microscopic scarring in tissue, damaging the genital system.
- Unrecognized, simmering genital-tract infections in men are massively common.
- If you've been hosting a guest infection for a long time, this will drag down your testosterone production and release.

WHAT TO DO

- Understand the issues around microbial infections.
- Meet some of the microbes.
- Know the conditions.
- Cleanse yourself.
- Practice sexual hygiene.
- Follow up annually.

UNDERSTAND THE ISSUES AROUND MICROBIAL INFECTIONS

Sex involves many things, including the importing and exporting of microbes.

Whenever your penis interacts with an available vagina, mouth, or anus, you will be importing huge numbers of germs—bacteria, viruses, and fungi.

Even if you have been faithful to your current partner for years, this free trade does not stop happening. That's just the nature of the openings and of the fluids exchanged.

After each sexual encounter, your immune system keeps you from sensing these bugs and from letting them get out of hand—and most of the time you will not feel anything.

But know this: microscopic germ warfare is taking place after *each* sexual encounter.

> LOOK, JUST BECAUSE you love someone, doesn't mean they are germ free. Affection can lead to infection.

Huge numbers of men get germs that cause *active* infections—the infections that you feel, with actual symptoms.

About 10 million men in North America get sexually transmitted diseases (STDs) every year. These are the men who actually feel their infection, come to doctors, and get treated. These are the men that we know about.

That's 10 million *new* cases annually.

One STD is chlamydia, an infection of *Chlamydia trachomatis*, a champion bacteria. This bug is the most common sexually transmitted disease in North America.

And even though 10 million infected men is a huge number, we estimate that there's an equal number of men—perhaps more—who get infections that nobody hears about, which are unrecognized and untreated. These are the men who get mild exposure to the bug and don't feel it at all.

And if they don't feel anything is wrong, they don't seek care, and this allows these softer invasions to simmer. But when the body contracts chlamydia, it goes to war. In fact, the body unleashes such intense firepower to kill this bug that even the heart can be affected, along with local testicular tissue. The home front (the testes) and the distant front (the heart) can both be damaged.

Now multiply this by how many other STDs are around.

Herpes

About 15 million men—*15 million*—have genital infections with the herpes simplex (aka herpes genitalis) virus right now.

It's a typical scenario: A man in his twenties had sex and then felt a vague genital discomfort but nothing terrible. Perhaps just one day of pain or burning or itching or tingling. But the feeling went away, so all must okay, right?

Wrong.

The men who actually feel a herpes infection are a small portion of the many more who become infected. Most of the time the infections are symptom free and "silent."

Generally, they did not feel anything when they got this infection initially.

So, of course, they haven't bothered to get any remedy, or to take any precaution to prevent the further spread of the virus.

And there are many other viruses that may also be present. (And we're not talking about the viruses that you hear about in the media, like HIV.)

Don't assume that just because you don't have any significant genital tract symptoms, you're germ free.

Infection Treatment Protocols Refer to Women Almost Exclusively

When women have infections, symptoms can be more noticeable or intense.

Yes, women do deserve special attention when it comes to sexually transmitted diseases. Because of their anatomy, they can have high-end complications, such as infertility due to scar tissue. They can also have intense symptoms that declare the infection—pain, discharge, odor, bleeding, and so on.

But it's almost never mentioned that, by the way, the man that she was having sex with, although he's not complaining of anything, likely *also* has the infection.

Treatment guidelines only talk about the man when the woman doesn't get better.

Current medical guidelines mention the male partner only when the woman keeps getting recurrent infections. When the doctors can't cleanse the woman, they *finally* realize that they might want to extend therapy to the man, too. All the while, of course, the man has been hosting the same infection.

And what happens if a woman is cured of a sexually transmitted disease with her first medication?

Then no one remembers about the man, and no one treats him. The woman is okay, she continues to have sex with her man, she doesn't seem to pick up the bug again, so the bug must be gone. Right?

Wrong.

The man generally will not feel the transmission of most bugs. Also, germs that enter via the penis have a habit of going up deep into the urinary system. So the infection *in the man* is just allowed to percolate, go deeper, take root, and continue the internal microscopic inflammation.

When treating infections, focusing on women only is a huge disservice to the delicate testosterone and sperm-producing tissues in the testes.

Oral Sex Transfers Germs, Too

Men have this idea that they can't get infections or bacteria or HIV from oral sex. Probably, they think, "It's not really sex, not really intercourse, is it?"

But the mouth actually has even more germs than the genitalia.

Men Damage Their Testicular Landscape Fighting Unrecognized Soft Infections

Mild exposure to germs, called subclinical infections, do not cause symptoms.

Let's say the man has just had vaginal sex, he's caught a few million germs in the backdraft, but feels no pain or problem. Now his immune system kicks in to clear the area. This is all happening under his radar, below his awareness, causing him no overt pain or discomfort at all.

As the immune policing system revs up, the cells in the testes that make testosterone get upset. These cells want to keep their neighborhood quiet. They don't want the biological equivalents of squad cars, attack dogs, the SWAT team, riot police, Tasers, investigators, and helicopters brought in.

But it's an issue of community safety, so the wishes of the local cells are overruled. Then all hell breaks loose.

When the infection clearing begins, like the clearing of criminals, a community-alert signal is sent out. It's like an air-raid siren, and local business slows or shuts down. Then there's a complete disruption of regular services and production, and resources get redeployed elsewhere.

Eventually, the immune police win. But they turn the place into a killing field. The cleanup operation leaves a pockmarked battle zone. The immune police have left many dead—enemy bugs, innocent bystanders, and their own police cells. There is debris, scar tissue, and scattered bullet holes everywhere, all cluttering the landscape, clogging blood vessels, irritating nerve insulation, and disrupting cell integrity.

This policing action by the immune system damages the delicate testosterone and sperm-producing cells of the testes. These cells are the innocent bystanders watching the police action helplessly.

Understand: this biological warfare happens under the man's radar, below his awareness, after *each* sexual encounter. And, because antibodies have memory, and remember how criminal bugs taste, the next armed response can be even more intense.

IF YOU LOOK under a microscope at tissue from which an infection has just been cleared, you can see the damage done by the immune police.

Depending on the strength and number of invading germs, the immune system mounts an intense attack. On a microscopic level, it looks like Hiroshima after the atomic bomb—a barren, deserted moonscape whose future growth has been stunted.

That's what happens to tiny parcels of land in the testes after even a mild exposure to germs.

So don't think you've been lucky if you have never experienced the symptoms of an STD. There may still be many kinds of germs—including those of STDs—quietly wreaking havoc, in battle with your immune system.

MEET SOME OF THE MICROBES

Here's a list of bugs to show you the range of microbes that you might be exposing yourself to. It is a subset of more than thirty common sexually transmitted diseases. These are the usual suspects that can cause noteworthy infections:

Chlamydia trachomatis

Even a slight itching around the penis might have been caused by this common bacteria.

It is difficult to identify, requires a special swab test, and even patients who get treatment are not retested to verify that the bacteria has been cleared. It can be cleared with high-powered antibiotics.

IN WOMEN, CHLAMYDIA causes scarring in the egg transport tubes. Silent brewing infections lead to PID, pelvic inflammatory disease. This is a major cause of female infertility.

Genital Herpes Simplex Virus

Symptoms can vary from a light prickling, tingling, or piercing sensation on the penis, to blisters, sores and ulcers. It is highly contagious, and can easily be transmitted through many routes—penile to vaginal, penile to oral, penile to anal, and penile to anything else you can think of.

It can even be transferred through oral sex from a person who has no actual sore on his or her mouth. There is no cure, only medications that control outbreaks.

Genital Human Papilloma Virus

Though this virus may cause warts on the penis, most infections are not recognized. It tends to stay external, on the skin, but can invade and cause genital cancers.

It is estimated that *half* of all men have had this virus at some point.

Because of the high rate of possible transmission, women always have to contend with the risks of contracting genital human papilloma virus. It leads to precancerous changes in the cervix, the opening of the uterus. This is the reason doctors recommend that women get annual Pap smear screening.

Chancroid

Little bumps, sores, and ulcers are caused by *Hemophilus ducreyi* bacteria. This organism also leads to swelling of the lymph glands in the groin. This condition is curable by antibiotics.

Gonorrhea

This infection usually declares itself, leading to yellowy-green pus discharge from the penis. This infection leads to pain on urinating and tender, painful testes.

Unrecognized or improperly treated infections can lead to colonization in the man's genital system, particularly in the prostate or at the top of the testes in the epididymis, the supercoiled tube that acts as a maturation stopover for sperm.

Meet More Germs of the Genital Landscape

When you ejaculate, your system opens up, and allows bugs to ascend into the genital tract. That is what is meant by the term *ascending infection.*

Here's just a partial list of microbes normally found in healthy vaginas. Most of these are part of the normal germ presence, the long-term guests who are stationed there, and who will be pleased to visit you, too:

Alpha-hemolytic Streptococci
Bacteroides ureolyticus
Candida albicans
Corynebacteria
E. coli
Enterococcus faecali
Fusobacterium nucleatum
Gardnerella vaginalis
Group B *Streptococci*
Klebsiella
Lactobacillus acidophilus
Mobiluncus
Mycoplasma hominis
Peptostreptococcus anaerobius
Peptostreptococcus prevotii
Peptostreptococcus tetradius
Prevotella bivia
Prevotella corporis

Proteus
Serratia
Staphylococcus epidermidis
Ureaplasma urealyticum

Where did all these germs come from?

It's mathematical. Let's say a partner is in a stable relationship. But before this, this person had sexual relations with five people. And those five people also had sexual relations with five people. And so on. Very quickly, you get into astronomical numbers.

So, in a microbiological sense, you are actually having sex not only with your current partner, but with all the partners that you both have had. And in your present relationship, you are contributing to your partner's germ landscape.

This is also how we breed superbugs. With so many bacteria mixing together, they talk, exchange DNA coats, borrow ingredients, teach each other new skills, learn each other's strengths, learn each other's language, share intelligence, and improve themselves.

These stronger bugs are harder to eradicate. They can survive in difficult terrain, and constantly look for new land to colonize.

So, the next time you and your partner have sex, and you think you're alone, remember that you also have a whole orchestra of accompanying germs. In fact, *more than three hundred* different organisms have been identified as part of the *usual and expected* contingent of genital microbes.

> **WHEN WE GRANDLY** list all these fancy-named bugs, we don't mean that there's only one or two of each of them in your partner.
> There are hundreds of thousands of each of these bugs, even millions. So you begin to get the idea of the exponential numbers of germs involved.

KNOW THE CONDITIONS

After sex, men may have some vague complaint—maybe some burning or discharge or irritation or skin itching or a lump or a bump. Men are thankful that most of the time these problems go away. But don't write it off until you get yourself checked out.

Just because the symptoms went away does not necessarily imply that the microbes disappeared. The microbes might have taken up residence at one of the drop-off stations in the male genital system.

After any sexual encounter, *any* discomfort should be investigated—even if it goes away. Don't give germs time to colonize your genital system.

These are areas where there may be the symptoms caused by germs in these guest houses:

Skin in the Genital Area

Skin in this area is often the anchor point, or entry point, for various infections. If you have any itching, irritation, rash, lump, bump, blister, or sore—especially if it started after a sexual encounter—have it investigated.

The Bladder

Urine is stored in the bladder for disposal. An infection here leads to pain, burning, and frequent urination. You may notice a profound change in the urine color, or even blood.

The Kidneys

These infections tend to be more serious, leading to fever, mid-lower-back pain, pain in the flanks, and groin pain. There can be urgent, painful, and frequent urination, and possibly even the passing of blood or a kidney stone fragment.

The Urethra

This is the tube coming from the bladder, through the prostate, through the penis to the outside. An infection here leads to pain and burning on urination, possibly also a discharge, depending on what organism is involved. The opening of the penis becomes red and irritated.

The Epididymis

This sits on top of each testis. It is a supercoiled tube that acts as a maturation stopover for sperm. An infection here leads to a swollen, painful scrotum that might make even walking difficult.

The Prostate

The prostate sits under the bladder. It adds fluid to the ejaculate that liquefies semen, making it more free-flowing. But the prostate also seems to be a wastebasket for junked germs.

Microbes often end up in the prostate, causing many symptoms. These include a deep groin pain, frequent and painful urination, even erection problems.

The Prostate

ABOUT 5 MILLION men in North America are treated for prostate infections every year. Even *more* men get prostate infections that go untreated.

Almost *half* of all men will get a prostate infection at some point in their lives.

Infections of the prostate are so complicated that doctors are running out of names. There is:

- Acute bacterial prostatitis (a short-lived infection of bacteria)
- Chronic bacterial prostatitis (a long-lived infection of bacteria)
- Acute on chronic bacterial prostatitis (a short-lived infection of bacteria, overlaid on a long-lived infection of bacteria)
- Asymptomatic inflammatory prostatitis (microscopic tissue irritation without the client feeling it—with no symptoms)
- Chronic nonbacterial prostatitis (a long-term prostate irritation with no known infectious cause)
- Chronic pelvic pain syndrome (ongoing genital pain that just lingers, without any traceable cause)

Some men will require antibiotics and other medications for months or even years.

CLEANSE YOURSELF

Do you have a secret infection?

Given the sexual practices of North American men, there's a 20 to 40 percent chance that you may have a previously undetected, hidden infection in the genital tract right now. Given this possibility, we recommend that you consider a round of cleansing antibiotics. Of course, this is best discussed with your health-care practitioner, and depends on things like how much unprotected sex (without a condom) you've had, and with how many different partners. So go and confess if you think you need to.

Doctors call this "treatment on spec"—cleaning you out on speculation.

Once doctors start looking, sometimes we do end up finding a number of hidden, low-grade chronic infections in the male genital tract. Depending on the findings, some men are offered one or more courses of antibiotics.

Don't Breed a Superbug

IF YOU HAVE more than one course of antibiotics, it should be a different antibiotic each time. If you let the bugs taste the same antibiotic each time, they learn how to outsmart the medication.

The bugs are intelligent and will adapt. Then the strongest microbes will emerge.

When doctors offer the same medication repeatedly, they unwittingly breed superbugs. This is part of the reason that so many germs are resistant to antibiotics.

There are also natural approaches to urinary and genital tract cleansing that you can do regularly. These include having lots of water, avoiding caffeine and alcohol, and drinking acidic liquids such as unsweetened cranberry juice (you can water this down for better taste). The acidic liquids act like pesticides, preventing microbes from making the genital tract their breeding ground.

These approaches can be used in addition to the antibiotic therapy recommendations, as needed.

EXAMPLE: You may be harboring *Chlamydia trachomatis*.
The antibiotic for this would be:

Zithromax (azithromycin), a single dose of 1 gram
or:
Doxycycline, 100 mg twice a day for 1 week

This and any subsequent course(s) of antibiotics can be decided with your health-care practitioner.

PRACTICE SEXUAL HYGIENE

Good sexual hygiene will protect your T-resources.

Condoms

Certainly, for sex with a new or random partner, use a condom. These days, there is too high a chance of getting a significant infection to do otherwise.

Wash Your Hands before You Have Sex, including before You Masturbate

Our hands touch an infinite variety of bacteria and other germs during a normal day. Washing your hands thoroughly, or in a pinch using hand-cleansing gels (these have been shown to be less effective than soap and water), is recommended *before* sex, not just after.

If people knew how many germs they touch in a typical day, they would be more conscious of washing before *any* intimate contact.

We expose ourselves to germs by handling dollar bills (which are filthy), sliding our hands on staircase banisters, turning taps or pushing flush levers in public washrooms, touching payphones, pushing elevator buttons, turning public doorknobs, and shaking hands with people who are ill. We also transmit our own germs from one area of our body to another via our hands, particularly by touching our mouths and noses.

Drink Extra Water after Sexual Encounters

Extra water helps to cleanse the genital tract. The general goal should be to drink enough water to make the urine completely clear, colorless, and odorless.

> GO AHEAD, MAKE your day. Drink some unsweetened cranberry juice in honor of your past sexual partners.

After Sex, Get Up and Urinate

Do not fall asleep immediately after sex. Urinate first. This is your best chance to purge yourself of a portion of the germs introduced during sex.

And this applies to any form of sex—vaginal, oral, anal, or self-service. This includes after masturbation.

Treat Both *Partners if Either One Is Diagnosed with a Genital Tract Infection*

Here is a typical scenario:

A man's partner is diagnosed with a genital infection. The man says, "It's okay, doc. I had my test. They didn't find anything . . . I'm clear."

Wrong.

Our tests may not be sophisticated enough to pick up your present or a past partner's gift of bugs to you. For example, urinary tract infections are not detected if the concentration of bacteria is less than 10,000 per milliliter. That means, unless you have more than 50,000 bugs per teaspoon, our tests still would not even pick it up.

It's a good rule of sexual hygiene to assume that *both* partners have had germ exposure when one partner is diagnosed with an infection.

Treat both partners.

Sexual Hygiene Protects Fertility

Avoiding infections and germ exposure preserves the integrity of the delicate testicular tissues. For example, *Chlamydia trachomatis* and gonorrhea are particularly known to cause scarring of sperm-producing cells and sperm-carrying tubes.

FOLLOW UP ANNUALLY

- Get a urine test annually (at least).
- If you have been previously diagnosed with a sexually-transmitted disease, have a swab test taken of your urethra (the penile opening) periodically.

A urine test is a relatively rough measure of any bacterial or germ presence. It's not the best of tests, but it's easy, simple, and inexpensive. For these reasons, HMOs tend not to object to paying for urine tests.

The swab test is more focused, more sensitive, and can offer more information about the bugs' personality than a urine test can. It is recommended for men who have already been officially diagnosed with a sexually transmitted disease. It's part of the retesting, which is seldom done, to monitor the potential for persistent or recurrent infection.

Time and again, doctors will do a urine test incidentally—for an insurance medical exam, an immigration test, as part a health screen for an employment health test, and so on. And we will often find that a man has had a long-term urinary tract infection.

He will recall having had some vague symptoms of a genital tract infection only after we closely question him. He'll reply, "Yes, doc, I do remember having something like that."

But by finding the infection so late, and allowing the microbes to colonize his genital tract for months or years before coming to our attention, the man has allowed his T-producing tissue to potentially suffer.

What to Do if an Infection Is Found

If there is the slightest hint of infection, bacteria, infection-fighting police cells, blood, discharge, or anything unusual, follow it up. You may need a further dose of a clean-out antibiotic.

Some men benefit from having antibiotics that clear the genital tract once a year. The decision to do this would need to be discussed with your own health-care practitioner.

There are several considerations: the number of sexual partners—current and past, the number and severity of previously diagnosed sexually transmitted diseases, current symptoms, current sexual habits, and current test results.

Don't assume that because you don't feel anything in the genital or urinary system, you don't have any bugs—the microbes are much smarter and far more subtle than that.

> SEX IS LIKE sport fishing. Sometimes you have no idea what you might catch.

EXTERNAL WORLD—

YOUR MIND AND OUTLOOK

12

Background Questions

CONTINUE YOUR ASSESSMENT with this section. It's about how you inter-act with the world, and the effects on your mind and outlook. As before, rate yourself.

Think of your score rating—None, Mild, Moderate, or Severe—as how urgently you need to follow the recommendations in part 3. (For the full story, see appendices A, B, and C, but I recommend that you work your way through the book in the chapter order given.)

——— Your Changing Personality ———
(11 questions)

1. Do you blame others more?

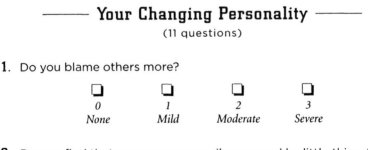

❏	❏	❏	❏
0	*1*	*2*	*3*
None	*Mild*	*Moderate*	*Severe*

2. Do you find that you are more easily annoyed by little things?

❏	❏	❏	❏
0	*1*	*2*	*3*
None	*Mild*	*Moderate*	*Severe*

3. Are you growing less tolerant of foreigners?

☐	☐	☐	☐
0	*1*	*2*	*3*
None	*Mild*	*Moderate*	*Severe*

4. Are you getting more difficult to get along with?

☐	☐	☐	☐
0	*1*	*2*	*3*
None	*Mild*	*Moderate*	*Severe*

5. Are you more grumpy and irritable?

☐	☐	☐	☐
0	*1*	*2*	*3*
None	*Mild*	*Moderate*	*Severe*

6. Have you become an injustice collector, cataloging the wrongs done to you?

☐	☐	☐	☐
0	*1*	*2*	*3*
None	*Mild*	*Moderate*	*Severe*

7. Do you have a shorter fuse, and blow up more frequently?

☐	☐	☐	☐
0	*1*	*2*	*3*
None	*Mild*	*Moderate*	*Severe*

8. Do your loved ones wonder why you're more resentful and hostile?

☐	☐	☐	☐
0	*1*	*2*	*3*
None	*Mild*	*Moderate*	*Severe*

9. *Is this you?* "I find myself feeling insulted more easily."

☐	☐	☐	☐
0	*1*	*2*	*3*
None	*Mild*	*Moderate*	*Severe*

10. Do you find yourself wishing revenge on your enemies more often?

☐	☐	☐	☐
0	*1*	*2*	*3*
None	*Mild*	*Moderate*	*Severe*

11. *Is this you?* On the road, another driver cuts in front of you. Your temper flares, you rage, shout insults, give him the finger, and wish you could nuke the guy off the face of the earth.

❏ ❏ ❏ ❏
0 *1* *2* *3*
None *Mild* *Moderate* *Severe*

Your Changing Personality

Your score:_____ / 33 points

Score/Rating
0 to 3   *None*
4 to 13   *Mild*
14 to 26 *Moderate*
27 to 33 *Severe*

——— Your Mind ———
(6 questions)

1. Is your thinking not as sharp, not as clear?

❏ ❏ ❏ ❏
0 *1* *2* *3*
None *Mild* *Moderate* *Severe*

2. Do you feel less creative, stuck for new ideas?

❏ ❏ ❏ ❏
0 *1* *2* *3*
None *Mild* *Moderate* *Severe*

3. *Is this you?* "I notice some difficulty from time to time searching for the right word."

❏ ❏ ❏ ❏
0 *1* *2* *3*
None *Mild* *Moderate* *Severe*

4. *Is this you?* "I find that learning new information is more of a struggle."

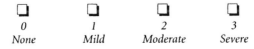

0 *1* *2* *3*
None *Mild* *Moderate* *Severe*

5. *Is this you?* "I find that I'm less able to figure things out, less able to analyze problems. I'm slower on the uptake."

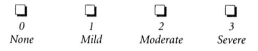

0	*1*	*2*	*3*
None	*Mild*	*Moderate*	*Severe*

6. *Is this you?* "I considered myself a pretty good thinker. But I'm not as decisive as I was before, and my attention span is shorter. I wonder if my memory is weakening."

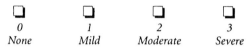

0	*1*	*2*	*3*
None	*Mild*	*Moderate*	*Severe*

Your Mind

Your score:_____/ 18 points

Score/Rating
0 to 2   *None*
3 to 7   *Mild*
8 to 14   *Moderate*
15 to 18 *Severe*

Consider your score ranges here for the questionnaires Your Changing Personality and Your Mind—did you score None, Mild, Moderate, or Severe? Your scores here will help you determine how urgently you need to follow the recommendations in part 3. These chapters are about stress levels, therapeutic self-massage, the workplace, relationships, and spirituality and health.

13

Stress Levels

LISTEN TO SOME men under stress:

"We've been married fifteen years, and sure we had some good times. But I guess we just grew apart. We were always arguing—it didn't really matter about what, big things, small things, anything really.

"Now I'm going through discovery proceedings for divorce. My lawyer tells me that half our marital assets will be split down the middle . . . and you know what? She is probably going to get our house. I paid the mortgage off over twelve years, and she'll probably walk away with it.

"But what really hurts is the way my kids look at me. . . . What a mess I've made."

"I'm an aeronautical engineer, and we design aircraft engines for midsize jets. I have busted my butt for my company. I can't tell you the amount of overtime I've put in, but management is looking at us funny. Now we're worried.

"They are letting us go, like we are redundant. They still need engineers, but now they send the design plans to young PhDs in Russia, and they redraft the plans there. Sitting at computers in Russia . . . And how much do they pay them? Fifteen grand a year, with no benefits, nothing.

"Money is tight. We just moved to a newer house, and my second daughter will also be going to college next year. Do you have any idea how much college costs now? It's unbelievable. We are carrying credit charges, and between that and the mortgage, we're feeling the pinch. The bills keep piling up, and expenses keep climbing. My salary and compensation don't keep pace."

"Why wouldn't I be stressed? I get up at six A.M., leave the house at seven, grab breakfast on the go. I commute through killer rush hour, make it to work by eight o'clock, when we usually have our business day management meeting. ... I've got all these deadlines, responsibilities, and people I supervise. I'll have at least twenty-five or thirty e-mails that I have to reply to, and god only knows how many phone calls I get ... It feels like my brain's getting crowded out.

"Lunch is two coffees and a couple of cigarettes, plus maybe a muffin or pastry or something. ... When I get home at night, I'm not the greatest companion. I just want to be fed and left alone. I'll crash in front of the TV for a couple of hours and watch whatever's on ... that's how I chill out. Well, that and a few beers.

"I feel like I'm only one step ahead of it all catching up to me. Sure, I make good money. But sometimes I wonder, what am I doin' to myself?"

> **WHAT YOU THINK** about on a regular basis affects your biochemistry. So it's vital that learn to control your thoughts—don't let them control you.

——— Your Stress Levels ———
(9 questions)

1. *Is this you?* "I'm feeling the load of too many responsibilities, and they keep coming."

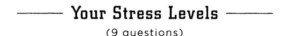

0	1	2	3
None	Mild	Moderate	Severe

2. Does your personality clash with that of your boss or supervisor?

0	1	2	3
None	Mild	Moderate	Severe

3. *Is this you?* "My home environment stresses me out frequently."

0	1	2	3
None	Mild	Moderate	Severe

4. *Is this you?* "The politics at work are such a headache."

0	1	2	3
None	Mild	Moderate	Severe

5. Do you often think, "Please, let me win the lottery so I can get the heck away from all that I have to deal with"?

❏	❏	❏	❏
0	*1*	*2*	*3*
None	*Mild*	*Moderate*	*Severe*

6. *Is this you?* "I would truly benefit from more regular vacation time."

❏	❏	❏	❏
0	*1*	*2*	*3*
None	*Mild*	*Moderate*	*Severe*

7. Do you feel like you're not performing at your best, and having more *off days*?

❏	❏	❏	❏
0	*1*	*2*	*3*
None	*Mild*	*Moderate*	*Severe*

8. *Is this you?* "To release stress, to relax, I'm turning to unhealthy practices—like drinking, smoking, or overeating. I know it's not good for me, but that's how I take the edge off."

❏	❏	❏	❏
0	*1*	*2*	*3*
None	*Mild*	*Moderate*	*Severe*

9. *Is this you?* "I often feel like I'm rushing from one activity to the next. I wonder if I'd qualify for this new condition they're talking about, 'hurried-man syndrome'?"

❏	❏	❏	❏
0	*1*	*2*	*3*
None	*Mild*	*Moderate*	*Severe*

Your Stress Levels

Your score:_____/ 27 points

Score/Rating

0 to 3	*None*
4 to 11	*Mild*
12 to 22	*Moderate*
23 to 27	*Severe*

Consider your score range here—is it None, Mild, Moderate, or Severe? Your score for the questionnaire Your Stress Levels will help you determine how urgently you need the recommendations here.

In the modern world, it's crucial to understand that perpetual stress poisons testosterone.

Follow the recommendations here to avoid letting stress get the better of you.

Key Points

- Chronic stress opposes testosterone.
- Testosterone opposes chronic stress.
- Men usually figure out that they are under chronic stress only when they get ill.
- Stress in men often shows up as hostility and irritability, not only depression.

WHAT TO DO

- Learn to recognize what chronic stress does to your body.
- Use short stress-control techniques for immediate needs.
- Learn the art of self-relaxation through guided imagery.

LEARN TO RECOGNIZE WHAT CHRONIC STRESS DOES TO YOUR BODY

Men under perpetual stress will develop many of the symptoms from this (partial) menu. The stress hormones cortisol and adrenaline (and other hormones) are responsible for these effects.

The Stress Hormones

Imagine you are asked to make a speech right now in front of a large group. You will momentarily feel the effects of the stress hormones cortisol and adrenaline.

These chemicals are helpful in short-lived situations, like making a speech, running for cover, or dealing with an immediate crisis. Whenever your body feels it's under attack or being challenged, these are the hormones that help you get through it.

Unfortunately, if you feel that you're under attack all the time—whether you're dealing with financial, marital, job, or family problems—these stress hormones don't turn off.

The nonstop flow of stress has many chemical effects in your body, one of which is the continuous release of cortisol.

And chronic cortisol overproduction dampens, neutralizes, and combats testosterone.

The Physical Effects of Stress

Chronic stress is a universal evil, aggravating, triggering, or worsening *all* other medical conditions.

For example, stress worsens joint pain, stomach burning, skin rashes, breathing problems such as asthma, migraine headaches, fertility problems, and so on.

- Blood pressure rises.
- Blood vessels tighten up.
- Your heart beats faster.
- Breathing becomes more shallow, taking in less oxygen.
- Sugar levels in the blood increase, released from liver storage.
- Fat levels in the blood increase, released from liver storage.
- Blood circulation is diverted to the brain and muscles—for you to run away, or to stand and fight.
- Blood circulation to internal organs, including the testes and penis, declines.
- Blood becomes more likely to clot.
- Sperm counts decline.
- Quality of orgasms declines.
- Many of the body's 700 muscles tighten up, leading to aches and pains.
- You are easily fatigued.
- Your appetite declines.
- You become restless, feeling trapped.
- You catch colds, coughs, and infections more easily, because resources are diverted away from the immune system.
- You get more canker sores in your mouth, again because the immune system is weakened.
- You develop sleep problems.
- You recover from illnesses more slowly.
- Your risk for cancer increases moderately.
- Your risk for heart attacks increases dramatically.

The Emotional Effects of Stress

Testosterone is involved in opposing all the following effects. When your T-levels aren't up to par,

- You lose interest in things that you enjoyed.

- You become emotionally unavailable and distant, unwilling to listen to your loved ones.
- You are easily annoyed.
- You become sarcastic and cynical.
- You feel anxious and on edge.
- You become irritable without provocation.
- You find it difficult to concentrate.
- You have too many thoughts to process.
- You feel like you're always behind in your schedule.
- You lose self-confidence.
- You lose your appetite for sex.
- You become hostile and negative.

The Physical and Emotional Effects of Stress Play off Each Other

It is important to understand that the physical effects of stress can cause emotional effects, and the other way around as well. This is a two-way street:

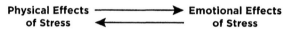

You can use this to your advantage to de-stress yourself. Ultimately, this is about using the power of your mind over your body, and the power of your body over your mind.

Replays, an Emotional Effect of Chronic Stress

ONE OF THE surest signs of chronic stress is having recurring, anxious, automatic thoughts. You keep dwelling on mistakes or setbacks. In your mind, you keep:

- Playing the same video over and over
- Reliving a negative conversation or encounter
- Repeating damaging self-talk
- Wondering again and again, "What is going to happen if . . . ?"
- Keep thinking up replies you should have given to someone who was confronting you

---

Recognize that this replay is a sign of stress, and adopt techniques to neutralize its many effects.

Stress control is a vast industry. There's yoga, Pilates, aromatherapy, writing letters to yourself, meditation, and so on. All these approaches have their devoted followers.

The following techniques described in this chapter work for my clients, who tend to be on the go and need ready, portable solutions, without many moving parts. While these exercises and techniques will seem foreign at first, once you incorporate them into your daily routine and get used to them, they will be quite helpful.

USE SHORT STRESS-CONTROL TECHNIQUES FOR IMMEDIATE NEEDS

Here are quick techniques for urgent needs—when you have a few seconds to a few minutes to de-stress.

Like learning any skill, practicing these techniques will give you stronger results over time. You will then òbtain more reliable and more robust relaxation.

Be Completely Still

Close your eyes and just *be*.

Stop everything that you are doing, physical movements as well as any thinking.

Turn your hypervigilance—your excessive preoccupation with your immediate circumstances—*off*.

Breathe deeply, holding your breath in for a second or two.

During this time, consciously have no goals, no deadlines, no pressing needs, nothing to be accomplished, no intruding thoughts.

As you practice this, you will find many of the physical changes of stress reverse—blood pressure, heart rate, and muscle tension are reduced. Shutting off thoughts clears and calms the mind.

Take a Deep Breath

Breathe as deeply as possible, with long, slow breaths, 5 to 12 times.

Breathe maximally.

As you take a giant breath in, *expand your chest fully, and inflate your stomach fully.*

Breathing is regulated by your automatic (autonomic) nervous system, along with your blood pressure and heartbeat. Consciously breathing deeply and slowly is like talking to your inner network, your automatic nervous system. This resets, downshifts, the pace of the body.

Do a Chin Tuck

Do the turtle:

Pull your chin in as far back as you can, like a turtle retracting its head back into its shell. Hold the retracted position for a few seconds. Do this five to twelve times.

This is a remarkably simple exercise which helps to release the muscle tension that builds up in the neck and upper shoulders. This is especially helpful for men who spend long hours sitting at a desk hunched over in the same position.

Do a Shoulder Roll

Make giant forward circles with your shoulders, moving them to their limits. Do this five to twelve times.

Again, this is a remarkably simple exercise which helps to release the muscle tension that builds up in the neck, upper back, and upper shoulders.

Reverse direction too, making giant backward circles with your shoulders, moving them to their limits.

Anyone who works at a desk, hunched over in the same position, should do this exercise a couple of times a day.

Pace

Pace around, walking back and forth in a single line, or following a circuit.

Walking helps you to work off energy and anxiety. The physical act of walking seems to demand attention from the body, taking it away from thinking about current stresses.

Many clients report that when they are faced with making major decisions, before important meetings, or before they go on stage to perform, pacing helps them deal with the stress.

Isolate Your Anger

Inevitably, you will lose control for some reason—you may be challenged, insulted, reprimanded, or ignored.

Instead of reacting with your *whole* body, learn to register the anger, tension, and rage with just your *right arm* or *right fist* (even if you are left-handed). Just let it tense up.

Don't hit anybody with the tensed-up fist—that's not the purpose.

By allowing your hand or arm to tense, you have given your body a valid outlet. You have not suppressed your anger, which has its own unhealthy consequences. This outlet is quiet, and mostly unnoticeable. It is also under your conscious control, and when you're done, you can let go, relax, and feel the rage disappearing from your arm.

If you focus the stress *only* to your right arm, you will notice that the rest of the body escapes having to go through a stress wave. Ultimately, this exercise will relax you, without causing any harm.

However, it's important to use the *right* arm, which is opposite your heart. If you use the left arm, some of the tension will be transferred to your cardiac system.

LEARN THE ART OF SELF-RELAXATION THROUGH *GUIDED THINKING*

Here are more elaborate stress-control exercises—for when you have at least fifteen minutes or more of protected time.

For these visualization techniques to work, you need to be sincere, to buy in to them. The material may sound hokey, New Age-y, unworkable, or weird. But give these techniques a chance. They are not psychological mumbo-jumbo.

In fact, these techniques are used in trauma care, cancer centers, burn care, heart surgery recovery, Olympic-class athletic training, team sports, high-performance racing, by doctors before giving certification exams, and by major corporations for senior management.

Basically, visualizations are like having a focused, directed, therapeutic daydream.

> SOME PEOPLE LIKE to have soft music or natural sounds, such as ocean or forest sounds, running in the background while doing these exercises.
> Whatever soft sounds add to your relaxation are welcome.

There are three scripts here. For each session, you need to be sitting or lying down comfortably in a quiet place where you will not be interrupted. For the scripts to work, you have to remove yourself from the everyday and fully open yourself to them. The scripts are only the triggering words—your imagination, intelligence, and ability to focus your mind will do the rest. Let yourself believe the scripts, and actually use your mind to *feel* the suggestions. Some clients repeat particular lines several times, to help them get into them. If you let yourself be transported by the words, you will actually feel the stress ebbing from your body.

The three scripts are:

- Hawaii relaxation
- Muscle-tension sweep
- Self-esteem (re)building

Fitting Relaxation into Modern Schedules

WE HAVE CLIENTS who carry these scripts on their handheld computers. They can then go through the script(s) whenever they have a few minutes to spare. Some have them typed on cards, which they carry in their wallets.

The Hawaii Relaxation Script

This sets up the sights, sounds, and feelings of a tropical paradise. You can read this out loud, or just to yourself, as you feel comfortable:

> *I am here on a gorgeous beach in Maui, one of the smaller islands of Hawaii.*
> *I can see the white sand glistening in the bright, bright sunlight.*
> *I can feel the warmth of the baking sand under my feet.*
> *A soft cool breeze stirs, just enough to take the edge off the Hawaiian sun.*
> *The air is fresh, perfumed, even tasty.*
> *Lush palm trees sway in the distance, and they are full of exotic colorful birds.*
> *The colors of everything are intense and vivid and delightful.*
> *I can hear soft music in the distance, and I can hear our picnic lunch being prepared.*
> *My body lotion has the fragrance of mango and coconut.*
> *I am feeling comfortably sleepy because of this cold Hawaiian fruit punch drink, with its crushed ice and fragrant tangy pineapple.*
> *All afternoon, I have been trying to count the waves as they reach the shore, slow and shimmering and endless—one by one they keep rolling in from the vast, open ocean.*
> *In the distance, I can barely see where the ocean ends and the sky begins.*
> *I can hear the surf lapping against the shoreline, slow and steady and peaceful.*
> *The waves bring in small shells, shiny and intricate. But I am too relaxed to pick one up.*
> *I don't need to be anywhere but here.*
> *I don't need to do anything except what I'm doing.*
> *This place is perfect.*
> *I feel calmness, a stillness, that is deep.*
> *I am at peace.*
> *I am me.*
> *I am worthy.*
> *I am special.*

The Muscle-Tension Sweep Script

This type of script is used in medical and dental schools for pain management, as well as by athletic trainers. Essentially, you create a feeling of active relaxation and healing in one part of your body, and then spread it.

Right Hand

I know that there is some tension in my right hand.
Slowly, I am letting this tightness, this spasm go.
I am letting my hand go limp.
I can feel relaxation going from my thumb and fingers to my palm, and down to my wrist.
My whole hand feels a little lighter and soothed.
If I were to visualize the relaxation going on in my hand, it's as if electricity were just flowing back and forth and in circles.
It's as if many beams of light were bouncing from one part of the hand to another.
I feel the hand is a little lighter, tingling, and relaxed.

Forearm to Elbow

As this feeling builds in my hand, it starts to radiate, flow, and spill upward into my forearm, up into my elbow.
Now the electricity is flowing from my fingertips to my elbow, back and forth and in circles.
It feels as if energy is bathing me from the inside.
With each wave the arm feels a little more relaxed, as if it's pleasantly asleep.
The muscles of my arm are loosening.

Right Shoulder

Now the feeling of relaxation and calm spreads into my right shoulder. The whole shoulder is losing its tension.
I can feel this.
The tightness and spasm is lifting.
Now the electricity is gently flowing from my fingertips up past my elbow, up to my shoulder, and back to my fingertips.
The relaxation is flowing back and forth and in circles.

Left Shoulder

The feeling of calm and energy now spreads from my right shoulder across to my left shoulder.
I can feel how my body eases out the tension and tightness.

Left Arm to Fingertips

The electricity, the beams of light, now continue to flow onward.
Down from my left shoulder, into my left elbow, into my left hand, all the way into the fingertips.
The easing of tension continues, and the warmth and tingling flow back and forth across my arms and shoulders.

Upward from Fingertips to Neck

*Now the energy flows up from the fingertips of both hands, up
past both elbows, past both shoulders, into the back of the neck.*

*I can feel my neck readjusting posture, letting go of tension, let-
ting the spasm fade away.*

*It's like electricity, beams of light, flowing from the fingertips all
the way to the back of the neck.*

*The energy flows back and forth, and with each pass the muscles
feel lighter.*

To the Forehead

*The tingling and relaxation now move up the neck, over the head,
all the way to the forehead.*

I can feel so much tension and muscle spasm just loosening.

*I can feel the energy flowing in the whole circuit, from the finger-
tips, to the arms, the neck, to the head, to the forehead.*

Down the Forehead to the Neck

The electricity now cascades down the forehead.

The eyes feel calm and relaxed and free of tension.

*The release continues down past the nose, into the muscles of the
face and cheek, down into the front of the neck.*

I feel a stillness and calm in all these areas.

*I can feel wave after wave of relaxing electricity flow from my fin-
gertips to the shoulders, to the neck, to the forehead, and down
to the front of my neck.*

It feels as if the energy is bathing me from the inside.

*I can sense the energy flowing over this whole circuit, back and
forth and in circles.*

Down the Chest and Down to the Middle Back

The electricity and energy flow downward.

Down the front of the chest, and down to the middle back.

*I can feel the warmth and tingling and lightness over the chest
and to the middle back.*

*I can feel the waves starting at the fingertips going through the
full circuit, past the neck, over the head, to the bottom of the
chest and the middle back.*

I feel a sense of peace and harmony in all these areas.

Down the Abdomen, and Down the Lower Back to the Hips

*The relaxation continues to flow, down the abdomen in the front,
down the lower back, and into the hips.*

*I can sense the beams of light traveling from the fingertips up the
arms, around the head, and downward to the chest and back,
right to the hips.*

I can feel the whole circuit active.

I can feel the whole circuit calm and relaxed.

*I can feel my lower back responding, readjusting, losing its
tightness.*

To the Knees

The relaxation continues to flow down the thighs to the knees.

*I can feel the knees readjusting, letting go of tension, letting the
spasm fade away.*

*Electricity and warmth and a tingling are now traveling this
whole circuit, again and again, from the fingertips, to the arms,
to the shoulders, to the neck, over the head—down, down
through the chest and lower back, to the hips, to the knees.*

The whole circuit is alive and activated and soothing.

To the Toes

*The electricity and relaxation flow from the knees down the legs,
past the ankles, into the tips of the toes.*

*I can see the beams of light traveling this whole circuit over the
whole body.*

*Again and again as each wave passes, the body feels less tension,
less stress.*

I feel calm.

I feel stilled.

I feel like I'm floating.

*I am letting these waves of relaxation wash over me again and
again.*

Visualization Is a Powerful Technique

TO ASSIST WITH conventional treatment for cancer and HIV,
scripts such as these are being used successfully to direct attention to regions of the body, even to particular organs.

Muscle-Tension Sweep Without the Script

After some rehearsal and using this script a few times, you will learn the
relaxation pathway described. Then you will not need the script word for
word. You will then be able to regenerate a feeling of calm, starting with your
right hand, and to spread that calm throughout your body at will.

Remember, the power of this progressive self-relaxation script depends on the power of your thinking, how intensely you can feel what the words suggest. If you just read it flat, it will do little for you.

Once you master this script, you will be surprised at how quickly you can start the relaxation in your right hand, and how quickly you can recruit other parts of the body to fully relax.

In fact, people report that once they have learned the scripts well, they find themselves automatically going through them—as if the body decides for itself when it needs to de-stress.

The Self-Esteem (Re)Building Script

This script helps you to move away from negative influences. Read it aloud or read it silently to yourself, as you see fit. If you trust someone enough, you can have him or her read it to you—this can be very powerful (they should change the *I* to *you*, of course).

Reading these lines quickly, without experiencing them, will make them sound like mere platitudes, like a greeting card. Let each line *mean* something to you. For example, when you read, *I know the good in me*, spend several seconds summoning up positive memories that reinforce this.

> *I have been through a great deal . . . many challenges . . . many*
> *   struggles . . . and many battles.*
> *I have weathered so many storms.*
> *And I am still standing.*
> *Others have tried to take me down.*
> *Others have tried to undermine me.*
> *Others have tried to take things away from me.*
> *I have made mistakes.*
> *But I am still standing . . . still with my pride . . . aware of my*
> *   own dignity.*
> *Many have tried to influence me.*
> *Some have disappointed me*
> *All my decisions have not been perfect.*
> *All my actions have not always been positive.*
> *But I have overcome them all.*
> *I have not always been good to my body.*
> *I have not always been good to my mind.*
> *I have not always been good to my spirit.*
> *But I am always hopeful.*
> *I am optimistic and confident.*
> *I deserve contentment.*
> *I deserve peace.*

I deserve tranquility.
I have earned it.
I can feel the light within.

I know the good in me.
I know the positive in me.
I know that I can strive to do better.
I know that I can strive to be healthy.
I know that I can use my intelligence.
I know that I have great capacity.
I know that I have many abilities.
I know that I can make my life better.
And I deserve success.
I deserve my share of victories.
I am ready for contentment.
I am ready for more happiness.
I am worthy of respect.
I am worthy of esteem.
I am worthy of affection.
I am worthy of love.
I am worthy of being cared for.
I deserve to be cherished.
I am worthy of being treasured.
I deserve to be valued.
I am worthy of being appreciated.
I deserve to stand tall.
I know the light within me.
I am content with myself.
I am pleased with myself.
And I am getting better all the time.
I am uniquely me.

DO NOT UNDERESTIMATE the power of this formalized self-talk, once it is practiced regularly.

Some people have described these scripts as "prayers for the modern man."

Shopping Therapy for Stress Control

BUYING AND SHOWING off gadgets leads to T-surges in men, and helps to control stress.

When men buy new toys, something special happens to them. When they go looking for the latest in stereo components, cell phones, DVD players, digital cameras, laser printers, microprocessors, color monitors, hard drives, laptops, satellites, or plasma or high-definition large-screen TVs—their testosterone level rises. The same applies if they are buying automobile components or home hardware like saws, drills, woodworking tools, and carpentry equipment—whatever they're into.

When men purchase these items, they feel cool, pleased, invigorated, elevated, current, and important. They feel as if they're buying a piece of magic. They think, "Wow, check this out. This is the best thing around. This is serious, and I deserve it.

Showing the item off also leads to a separate testosterone surge. When men see the look of envy in their friends' eyes as they're displaying their new toy, they get a hormonal spike. The awed admiration of their friends feeds their T-chemistry. And this can happen each time they show the item off.

Men feel they have bettered their friends and outdone them. They use competitive language, talking about how their gadget is bigger and has faster speed, higher capacity, greater resolution, or a next-generation component. Men will brag about the size of their hard drive, the speed of their processor, that they are wireless, networked, or at the cutting edge of technology. They will even brag about how good a deal they got, showing off their financial wizardry.

This T-connection is perhaps the underlying reason why men purchase hardware way beyond what they *need*. This is part of the chemical explanation of conspicuous consumption. In fact, showing off electronics can actually lead to larger T-spikes than when men were just purchasing the gadget.

14

Therapeutic
Self-Massage

"**L**OOK, DOC, I'M** ready to follow your program. But you want me to do *what?* . . . You're serious?"

Yes.

This is a wake-up call. Pay attention to the environment you make the testes live in. You drag them around all day, all bottled up, never bothering to think what they might like, and never paying attention to what helps or hurts them. Then you want the testes to come up with the goods on demand, whenever and wherever you want to have sex. And then when they're back under cover, not to be consulted again. What kind of treatment is this? No wonder you may be feeling sluggish.

Follow the therapeutic self-massage recommendations here to increase your drive, maximize your T, and lead to many other health benefits. Then you will better appreciate the wisdom contained in the immortal words of John Wayne: "If you've got them by the balls, their hearts and minds will follow."

But first, take this questionnaire to determine your present drive.

—— Your Drive ——
(10 questions)

1. Are you less enthusiastic about *home* activities and projects that used to stir your imagination?

☐	☐	☐	☐
0	*1*	*2*	*3*
None	*Mild*	*Moderate*	*Severe*

2. Are you less eager about *work* activities and projects that used to stir your imagination?

☐	☐	☐	☐
0	*1*	*2*	*3*
None	*Mild*	*Moderate*	*Severe*

3. When completing a task or project, do you settle for what's adequate, not for the best that you can do?

☐	☐	☐	☐
0	*1*	*2*	*3*
None	*Mild*	*Moderate*	*Severe*

4. *Is this you?* "I'm not so motivated to take on new challenges. I'm comfortable in my settled ways."

☐	☐	☐	☐
0	*1*	*2*	*3*
None	*Mild*	*Moderate*	*Severe*

5. *Is this you?* "I don't feel so ambitious at work anymore. I feel blocked."

☐	☐	☐	☐
0	*1*	*2*	*3*
None	*Mild*	*Moderate*	*Severe*

6. *Is this you?* "I'm not as self-confident as before."

☐	☐	☐	☐
0	*1*	*2*	*3*
None	*Mild*	*Moderate*	*Severe*

7. *Is this you?* "I pursue fewer social engagements and make fewer good friends now."

☐	☐	☐	☐
0	*1*	*2*	*3*
None	*Mild*	*Moderate*	*Severe*

8. *Is this you?* "Before, I felt like I had four-wheel drive. Now, I'm not so sure."

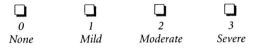

☐	☐	☐	☐
0	1	2	3
None	Mild	Moderate	Severe

9. *Is this you?* "I do live with the possibility of losing my job, of being downsized. It can be quite disheartening."

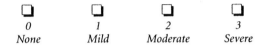

☐	☐	☐	☐
0	1	2	3
None	Mild	Moderate	Severe

10. At work, do you think, "God, how many more years do I have to do this?"

☐	☐	☐	☐
0	1	2	3
None	Mild	Moderate	Severe

11. *Is this you?* "I feel somewhat intimidated by the younger guys at work. It's like they're ready to take over, to displace me. That saps your dedication."

☐	☐	☐	☐
0	1	2	3
None	Mild	Moderate	Severe

Your Drive

Your score:_____/ 30 points

Score/Rating
0 to 3   *None*
4 to 12   *Mild*
13 to 24   *Moderate*
25 to 30   *Severe*

Consider your score range here—is it None, Mild, Moderate, or Severe? Your score will help you determine how urgently you need the recommendations in this chapter.

Like many men, you probably believe the genital region is only there for sex. But massage will soothe, awaken, and fortify the area with results that will recharge your entire body.

Key Points

- Massage soothes, awakens, and fortifies a body area.
- Men only pay attention to their genital region for sex.

$$\boxed{\textbf{WHAT TO DO}}$$

- Keep the testes at the temperature they want to be kept at. Avoid pelvic and genital heat.
- Sit properly—from the testes' point of view. Do V-checks throughout the day.
- Self-massage the testes and perineum.

KEEP THE TESTES AT THE TEMPERATURE THEY WANT TO BE KEPT AT. AVOID PELVIC AND GENITAL HEAT.

Both you and your testes need to stay cool.

How Sensitive Are the Testes to Temperature?

IT MAY TAKE the testes up to three months to fully recover from one day of fever.

Now that's delicate.

A Privileged Position in a Gated Community

Testosterone is not stored anywhere in the body. It is not banked. Remarkably, in this respect, it is unlike almost any other substance the body makes, including the equivalent female hormone, estrogen.

The body thinks T is nuclear. It considers T too powerful to store in quantity—too powerful to let you have immediate access to any stockpile. This is why T is made fresh, round the clock, continuously.

The testes and their prized products—sperm and testosterone—are too important to be left inside your body, and too important to trust you with them. They reside in their own special zone.

To brew testosterone and assemble sperm, the testes want their own environment, their own temperature setting, and they screen all visitors, intruders, and foreign elements.

Hear this: the testes hang within a free-floating sac, the bag called the scrotum. Why? Because they were meant to fly free and swing in the breeze. Specifically, to keep the testes working at their best, you have to keep them about 6 degrees Fahrenheit below your own core body temperature.

Six degrees is huge. You can feel a six-degree difference. That's the difference between, say, a comfortable room temperature of 75 degrees Fahrenheit, and an oppressive 81 degrees. In fact, each batch of testosterone and sperm is monitored for quality-control purposes. Heated testosterone or sperm does not pass the testes' own quality-control tests.

Heat damages both T-output and sperm production. In fact, hot-tub temperatures cause the testes to send out a little mini-grenade called a heat-shock protein. It's as if to say, "Sorry, all the testosterone and sperm that we were working on just now won't be shipment quality, retail grade. We're throwing them out or holding back a bit."

When a couple complains of infertility, and it's found that the man has a low sperm count, cooling the testes is one of the first recommendations made. In fact, problems in men now account for the majority for fertility difficulties.

In our society, however, we arrange everything to challenge this testicular temperature request. The testes try to forgive us, try to accommodate us, but they can't.

You need to better accommodate them. As much as possible,

- Avoid Using Car Seat Heaters. Higher-end cars come equipped with seat heaters, which in some cases go on automatically in cold weather. During winter in North America, the snowbound among us turn these heater switches on and leave them on. For months. We, along with our testes, bake. Similarly, if you live in a hot climate, your car seats will absorb the sun's heat. When you return from an afternoon of shopping, you can be sure that the heat is being transmitted to your pelvic area.

Also, as much as possible,

- Avoid taking hot-tub and hot whirlpool baths.
- Avoid heated water beds. Water beds can raise testicular temperature by almost 10 degrees Fahrenheit.
- Avoid using electric blankets.

In addition,

- Cool down the water temperature when taking a shower.
- If you have a movable showerhead, especially with pulsating massage, do not use hot water directly on your genital region.
- When you come out of the shower, wear a bathrobe for at least thirty to forty-five minutes before you dress.

- Avoid tight, restrictive clothing, like tight jeans, designer underwear, or underwear made of nylon or wool.
- Wear loose-fitting cotton boxer shorts.
- Wear pants that are loose fitting, preferably with front pleats, which have extra room for your equipment.

CHILDREN'S SPECIALISTS ARE noting that baby boys who for years wear disposable diapers, which are sealed by light plastics, may be damaging their testosterone and sperm production. The plastics seal in heat.

They recommend old-fashioned washable cotton diapers that breathe.

It seems that the scrotum is happiest naked. That's probably best, if you can swing it. But, assuming that walking around naked may not be appropriate for too long in your home, you might wish to wear a terry-cloth robe.

Give the testes some freedom. The point here is to avoid the constant constraint of pants, pajamas, briefs, or track pants. The testes themselves have only the thinnest layer of skin over them, and they don't appreciate your putting on extra layers.

The testes and scrotum do their climate assessment, their weather check, all the time. And the brain acts on that assessment about every fifteen minutes, telling the testes to make more T, or withhold it, as necessary.

Wearing the robe for at least thirty to forty-five minutes lets at least two or three brain orders come in, with the testes unconfined.

If you don't like robes, just wear a towel, with the knot tied on your side at your hips. Incidentally, that's how most men in high-sperm, very fertile Eastern countries walk around *all the time*—open and ventilated. In fact, sperm counts are rising in such third world countries, whereas counts in the Western world have declined by 50 percent in the last forty years.

Scottish men, with their kilts, were onto a dress code that fostered T-effects. When Mel Gibson shouted "Freedom!" in the movie *Braveheart*, maybe he was speaking truer than he knew. He might also have been celebrating kilts, which keep the testes free. And there's the old gag, "What does a Scotsman wear under his kilt?" The implication, of course, is that *real* Scotsmen don't wear anything.

Don't Use Laptop Computers on Top of Your Lap

This will burn you guys where you don't want.

Depending on the model, processor, and cooling fan in your computer, a laptop can increase your groin and scrotal temperature by anywhere from

1 to 5 degrees Fahrenheit. Take a moment to feel the heat a laptop gives off; you may be surprised.

With prolonged exposure, the laptop heat can damage the testosterone production facilities to the point where sperm are deformed, weaker, and give up their quest easily. This way, for sure you will not produce as many good long-distance swimmers.

Don't watch a DVD movie, play a virtual game, or word process with the computer directly on your lap. Period.

Wash or Wipe the Testes with Moderately Cool Water Two to Three Times a Day

Ever used cool water to soothe your eyes? Tea bags? An ice-pack gel?

The testes would like a little bit of catering, too.

Now, we know that sounds bizarre. Men look at us like we're mad when we counsel them to do this. But by late afternoon, many men have been sitting for hours. They've been generating and trapping groin heat. Things are sweaty, which is your body's and testes' way of telling you that that area is too hot. It is part of the reason that T-levels are lowest in the late afternoon.

GOODNESS, YOU MEN are so concerned about sweat in your underarms. Fine, you don't want to scare your neighbor, so you're willing to spend billions on sweat and odor control.

But I can assure you that your underarms do *nothing* for you. It's just dead space.

When the testes sweat, the body's going to hear about it, even if you don't. So help them out a little.

Whether at home or in the washroom stall, wipe your testicles with comfortably cool water, letting them enjoy the coolness for about fifteen seconds at least. Wipe away the sweat and let the area breathe.

Many men—though not all—report that washing their testes with cool water ten to fifteen minutes before sex enhances the experience. Try it.

Do not use ice cubes. Eager clients want to follow advice, and think, "If cool water is good, super ice cold must be better." Wrong.

SIT PROPERLY—FROM THE TESTES' POINT OF VIEW

Much has been written about ergonomics, about seat design and the correct way to sit. How to keep your back straight with special supports, how to avoid hand fatigue with wrist rests and special mouse pads, the correct forward sloping angle, where to sit on the seat, and so on.

Nothing is ever mentioned about the testes, which take slow revenge if they're allowed to bake under squished pressure.

Consider the way you might be sitting right now. If your legs are reasonably close together, they squish the scrotum, trap heat, put pressure on the blood going into and coming out of the scrotum, dampen nerve impulses, and don't let the area breathe. Sitting with your legs comfortably together raises the scrotum temperature by almost 4 degrees Fahrenheit.

You think the standard yoga lotus position, with legs wide apart, far away from the testes, is a coincidence?

Possibly, but it's ergonomically sound from the testes' point of view.

Unfortunately, for North American males, sitting is what we do best. At meetings, in the car, at the dining table, watching TV, at work, at school, at restaurants, at movies, at worship services, while reading the newspaper, listening to radio, in front of your computer, while on the phone, on air flights, on subways and buses, in stadiums and arenas, for haircuts, and—of course—waiting for your health-care practitioner.

For six out of ten men, that's all you do. No exercise whatsoever. We just move to change our sitting locations from place to place.

Leg gone to sleep?

We've all had the experience. You've been sitting on the ground for a while, maybe with one leg folded under your buttocks.

You get up and your leg is asleep. You have numbness and tingling and you can't move it. Your leg won't accept your weight yet. You shake it, and you have to wait a minute or so before it wakes up.

This happens because pressure was put on the nerves and circulation. Everyone has experienced this and knows the feeling.

The same thing on a softer scale goes on all the time in the testes because of poor sitting habits and prolonged sitting.

Do a V-Check

When you sit, your legs make a V. When you know you will be sitting anywhere for more than fifteen minutes, consciously try to sit with your legs further apart to make a wider V.

With enough space, there will actually be some breathing room for your testes on either side of the scrotum. That's what you want. This position avoids the heat trapping, the squishing, the circulatory pressure, the challenge to the nerve impulses, and allows for better outgoing drainage. This is environmental control for the testes.

Now, there are considerations as to how far you can sit with your legs apart and still look appropriate. If your legs are hidden under a desk or tablecloth, there's no problem. If you're on a sofa at a formal meeting or sitting on public transportation, you may not wish to spread your legs and look like a big dumb jock, or like your knuckles drag ape style.

Even so, try to make a wide V every so often, and keep your legs further apart than usual. Moving your legs around like this also helps the general circulation into and out of your legs, too. Don't get obsessive about it. Every few minutes or so is enough.

SELF-MASSAGE THE TESTES AND PERINEUM

"You want me to *play* with myself?"

No, not in this chapter. This is just testicular maintenance, although it does sound unusual.

The laying on of hands, therapeutic massage, is basic to the practice of health care. If you have a headache, tense shoulders, neck strain, or pain in the bottoms of your feet, a well-applied massage soothes and relaxes.

We naturally massage parts of the body that call to us, that announce their fatigue, aching, or tiredness. But we very seldom massage for enhancement.

Where Is Your Perineum?

When you sit on a bike or on a horse, you're sitting on your perineum. It's the underside area of your body from the front of the anus to the beginning of your scrotum.

Men who sit repeatedly and for too long on bicycles with typical "banana" seats damage their perineum. The damage is to both the circulation and nerve wiring.

This can lead to diminished T-effects, including decreased sperm count, infertility, and erectile dysfunction.

The main cable involved is called the pudendal nerve. This supplies—talks to—the prostate gland, the penis, and the scrotum.

In women, this nerve supplies—talks to—the clitoris.

Remember, the Testes Are Incredibly Sensitive

If you want to hurt a man, the classic thing to do is to "kick him in the balls."

Why is this so efficient? Because the area in and around the underside of the testes is one of the most sensitive parts of a man's body. There are a huge number of nerves, coiled arteries and veins, in multiple, crisscrossing pathways.

In short, this is a high-resolution, high-fidelity, surround-sound area for a man. A kick here gets a strong message to him good and quick.

We can exploit this extraordinary sensitivity for your benefit. Here's how.

> BY THE TIME YOU'RE forty years old, you've probably brushed your teeth twenty-five thousand times. Would you mind letting the testes get in on some of that action?

Perineal Massage

With a tissue in hand, stroke the perineal area, going from *back to front*, from in front of your anus to the underside of your scrotum.

Do this anywhere from one to three times per day, fifty strokes each time (*yes*, fifty).

All right, how's this going to work? First, start from a standing position and squat down somewhat. Open your legs up to give you access. Some men may need to support themselves.

Hold a tissue as if you were going to wipe your mouth. With the folded tissue paper in hand, use quick, mild pressure in forward motions. It's more than a tickle.

The fifty strokes should take about sixty seconds in total—just one minute. Let the testes jiggle in the air as your hand comes forward, stroking the underside of your scrotum.

If you're taking longer than sixty seconds, you're doing something too kinky or too forceful. Leave the penis alone. If you arouse yourself, you'll use up the T, actually spend it, as it's produced.

> ### Cautions
>
> MAKE SURE YOUR nails are trimmed. Men have drawn perineal or scrotal blood with unexpected snags on fingernails.
>
> Also, don't do the massage too vigorously, or you can get chafing of the skin on the underside.

Understand, this is a nonsexual, self-applied mini-massage therapy. It's chiropractic for the private parts, physiotherapy for the scrotum, kinesiology for T-production. It is based on sound principles of human physiology, medicine, and therapeutic massage—even if it sounds peculiar.

Why Self-Massage the Testes and Perineum?

With time, this massage increases blood flow to the important structures, builds extra blood vessels for more supply, and brings the nerves closer to the skin surface.

It increases the number of testosterone receptors in the nerves, vessels, and muscles. It speeds up nerve impulses, and makes the nerves fire more intensely. The reflexes get faster and more intense. The DNA in the genes gets switched on and makes more proteins. The whole system gets more responsive.

We're looking at full employment at full production capacity, with no lay-offs, and ISO certification. All of these increase T-impact across the body.

What Does It Feel Like?

Because there are so many overlapping nerves in this sensitive area, there are many layers of sensations. For example, if you do the same kind of stroking of your knee cap, it's a pretty straightforward sensation. Your body says, "Well, you're stroking our kneecap. So what?" That's because your kneecap has the basic, no-frills package of nerve fibers.

However, the perineum and underside of the scrotum are the exact opposite. They have the platinum deluxe package of nerves. You can feel the difference.

When you do the perineal massage, your body's systems say, "Okay, whatever you're doing, that's nice. It's like an inner tightness, a tingling, a pleasant spasm. Sort of what we feel in the lead-up to orgasm—refreshing, energizing, a wake-up. Even a heightened awareness."

One client commented, "It's like I'm teasing myself." That may in a sense be true, and may be partly what activates the area.

By doing this regularly, you are also communicating to your insides. This is what you as a man are saying to your own body's systems: "Look, the testicular environment is a priority area. I need this whole area activated, resourced, renovated, and juiced up. I apologize for the heat abuse and neglect. Send in a little more blood flow, please. Get those nerves, arteries, and veins fired up. Then the production of our chief exports—sperm and testosterone—should proceed much better."

Finding the Opportunity for Self-Massage

"C'mon, how am I supposed to drop my drawers, squat down, and pull a stunt like that?"

Good question.

Two opportunities during the day for this self-massage are in the morning when you're getting dressed, and in the evening when you're getting undressed.

But how will you perform this self-massage if you need to do it three times a day?

Men urinate anywhere from three to seven times during waking hours. (Any more than that may indicate problems such as diabetes or prostate gland enlargement.) My proposal is this:

When you have to urinate, whether you're at home or at work, urinate sitting down on the toilet.

Just sitting down, taking a load off, begins to relax the area. No more peek-a-boo peeing through your zipper only. When you're done, do the self-massage. You're already alone, exposed, and you have to stand up anyway. Before dressing fully, that's your opportunity.

Sometimes, go and visit the washroom stall to do the self-massage even when you don't have to urinate. Take a T-break. With these suggestions, you should be able to find time for this exercise during even the busiest days.

Don't Self-Massage During the Night

IF YOU GET up from sleep to urinate, do *not* do this self-massage at this time. It's energizing and might interfere with your getting back to sleep.

Do *not* do this self-massage more than three times in one day. It seems the body and the perineal area develop tolerance and don't respond with such delighted surprise if it's done too much.

Partners:

PLEASE REMIND YOUR man to do these exercises. He may not remember entirely on his own.

15

Workplace

"**T**ELL US ABOUT *yourself.*"
    If you ask a man to tell you about himself, he tends to talk all about his work, and only then gets to personal details.

He will discuss his current job, his title, his work responsibilities, his skills, how long he's had this job, the education he got along the way, even all the jobs he's ever held. Only after exhausting all that will he remember that he's a father or husband, or will he say anything about his home or life outside work.

If you ask a woman to tell you about herself, even if she has a high-powered job, *generally* she will talk about being a wife, mother, or grandmother much faster. She will bring up personal aspects far more quickly.

It seems to be the difference between how men and women define themselves. This is why it is important for you to understand how your career setting can influence and constrain your chemical profile.

─── Your Self-Esteem ───
(10 questions)

1. Do you feel what you contribute to your *household* is taken for granted, and not appreciated enough?

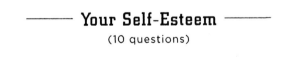

0	1	2	3
None	Mild	Moderate	Severe

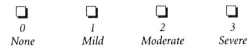

2. Do you feel what you contribute to your *workplace* is taken for granted, and not appreciated enough?

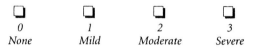

| 0 | 1 | 2 | 3 |
| None | Mild | Moderate | Severe |

3. *Is this you?* "I think there's less opportunity for me to advance now. This is making me bitter."

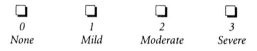

| 0 | 1 | 2 | 3 |
| None | Mild | Moderate | Severe |

4. Do you feel you are making less money than you're worth?

| 0 | 1 | 2 | 3 |
| None | Mild | Moderate | Severe |

5. *Is this you?* "I think that I have passed my peak."

| 0 | 1 | 2 | 3 |
| None | Mild | Moderate | Severe |

6. *Is this you?* "I thought I would own more by now."

| 0 | 1 | 2 | 3 |
| None | Mild | Moderate | Severe |

7. Is it important to you that your favorite sports team(s) win?

| 0 | 1 | 2 | 3 |
| None | Mild | Moderate | Severe |

8. Do your kids or colleagues joke that you are definitely part of the older generation?

| 0 | 1 | 2 | 3 |
| None | Mild | Moderate | Severe |

9. *Is this you?* "I feel that my contemporaries and colleagues get ahead and get promoted faster than me. I feel cheated."

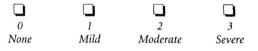

| 0 | 1 | 2 | 3 |
| None | Mild | Moderate | Severe |

10. *Is this you?* "You try and do right by your kids. You give them everything they need . . . love, everything. But what happens? I have to say, my kids disappoint me. They haven't lived up to my expectations."

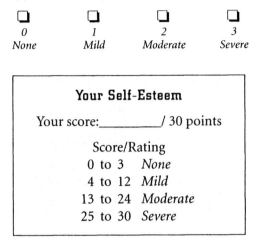

❑	❑	❑	❑
0	*1*	*2*	*3*
None	*Mild*	*Moderate*	*Severe*

Your Self-Esteem

Your score:_____/ 30 points

Score/Rating
0 to 3   *None*
4 to 12   *Mild*
13 to 24   *Moderate*
25 to 30   *Severe*

Consider your score range here—is it None, Mild, Moderate, or Severe? Your score will help you determine how urgently you need the recommendations in this chapter. In fact, it is said, "We are our work."

Your work setting affects your emotions, which in turn affect your hormones, including T. This is especially true for men, as their job is such an important defining element in their lives—perhaps the most important.

Follow the recommendations in this chapter to better navigate the workplace with this in mind.

A WORKPLACE ANALYSIS

THE EMOTIONAL TONE of where you work has a deep impact on the trend lines and spikes of your testosterone.

For many men, work is usually the main source of their self-identity—what they think of themselves, and how they think society views them. Work is where men get their ego boosted or smashed. And it's those ego boosts or letdowns that in turn get translated into upward or downward movements in your T-levels. It's as if T is a chemical marker of how your work day is going.

It is important for you to determine if the emotional environment at your workplace is positive, which will be protestosterone; or if it is negative, which will be antitestosterone.

It is also important to understand how your work setting can build up or drag down hormone effects on a long-term basis. Then you can prepare for potential negative experiences before you're in the middle of them.

Key Points
- Men who feel they are successful at work get more testosterone spikes.
- More testosterone spikes lead to more energy, drive, and success at work.

WHAT TO DO

- Understand how specific work issues affect you.
- Arm yourself against coworkers who may drag you down.
- Make sure you bond with your loved one(s) *daily*.

UNDERSTAND HOW SPECIFIC WORK ISSUES AFFECT YOU

Stability, Security of job

If you don't feel your job is secure, your T-releases are more fragile, muted, and dampened.

A fifty-two-year-old factory foreman said, "Doc, I don't know what's going on in this country. Do you know how many good-paying manufacturing jobs we've lost here? I could be phased out at any time. . . . They're sending all the jobs to Asia. If our union guys make any noise, they try to decertify the union. . . . If we get sold off to some other company, we lose all our protection, benefits, and contract rights. Out the window, gone. We have to start negotiating all over again, from scratch. There's no stability."

Unfortunately, too many men are living with the threat of layoffs, job loss, being downsized, company takeovers, having a younger guy in their company take their spot, or having their job exported to the third world.

This unsettled, unstable situation slowly bleeds men's T-responsiveness.

I realize that job stability is not easy to acquire on demand, and many men have little choice. But, as much as possible, work for a company or a division or a department or a branch that has stable prospects—that won't evaporate with two weeks' notice. Otherwise, your T-releases will be diminished, reflecting your lack of confidence in your current job situation. Then both you and your hormones live in a twilight zone.

One option for some men is to actively seek out a lower-paying but more secure job. Hormonally, that may be advisable, but you must tailor your decision to your own circumstances.

Feeling Valued by Your Co-Workers Enhances T

"The fellows I work with . . . they're like my family," says a forty-eight-year-old engineer who works in an auto engine design group. He describes their workflow as coordinated and respectful. They can have heated arguments about specific design elements, but they reach a team consensus before they present their ideas to management.

If you feel like you are a valued member of a team, that you're being relied upon to do your share, this builds your T-strength greatly. Being taken seriously boosts your ego, and this ups your T.

Cubicle Man

THERE'S A NEW species of man, called Cubicle Man. He sits in a cubicle, part of a huge corporate maze. He sits in isolation, lost in the system, just a cog in a machine. He does not feel respected, nor that his creative input is valued.

He has blunted T-spikes and his testosterone responsiveness fades with time.

This is precisely the type of man who will seek artificial boosts to his chemistry—smoking, drinking, devoting himself to spectator sports, even illicit drugs.

Dealing with Assaults on Your Self-Esteem

Because men make such an emotional investment in their jobs, being viewed negatively by co-workers can have lasting effects. This is an extreme example, but it does highlight some general points.

One client developed a disabling depression because of his co-workers. This was all because he was awarded a gag prize for the "messiest work area."

This client was a shop-floor maintenance crewman, one of five, in charge of making sure an aircraft assembly plant was in working order. He had worked for this same company for eight years and took pride in his job. At the annual Christmas party, he was stunned when he was given "the People's Choice Award for messiest work area."

He recalled the trauma: "I can still hear the laughter. I smiled the whole time. I wish I had just walked out, but I was too stupid . . . too shocked to think. I walked up to the front and accepted that son-of-a-bitch prize. I don't even want to tell you what it said on the card. And it was signed by everyone in my assembly group—*everyone* was in on it. They kept congratulating me for days. 'Way to go, couldn't have happened to a better man, a really deserving candidate.'

"I'm good at what I do. My wife is telling me to get over it . . . but it was humiliating. That day something snapped in me."

Your co-workers' opinion of you has real chemical effects on your system. You will feel the little rises or assaults on your self-esteem, which ultimately play out on your hormones.

Spread Some Sunshine

Actively cultivate friendship and favors with your immediate co-workers, team members, and office neighbors—even the ones you don't like. Consciously find things to praise and recognize people for, and they will think you're an excellent judge of character. Complimenting people makes them feel important. In fact, if you do this, you become a source of T-elevation for other men.

As much as possible, do not make enemies, because this will come back to haunt you in entirely unforeseen ways.

Feeling a Sense of Competence and Mastery in Your Job Enhances T

Knowing what you're doing, and then being given the opportunity to shine, is very sustaining to the male hormone. Exercising skills that you have mastered activates the brain on multiple levels. You can recognize this sense of competence when you hear a man proudly saying, "I'm *doing* what I was *trained* to do."

One of my clients is a forty-one-year-old garbage collector working for a large city. He enjoys his work, says he's making good money, and that his three-man team work together like a tuned machine.

He's the "curb guy," which means he's the one closest to the curb, signaling to the garbage-truck driver when to load, and when to move on. He prefers to pick up round garbage barrels, leaving cardboard boxes and odd-sized packages for his loading partner. This is all by prearrangement, silently understood when they're out on the street.

If the load is too heavy for the two men, the driver will get out and help, even though that's not his responsibility. This garbage collector describes his work with pride, as if it's choreography from a fine ballet.

So the T-spikes and trend lines have more to do with how you *feel* about your job than with how elevated your job actually is.

Acquire Competence to the Point of Mastery

What's fascinating from a chemistry point of view is that it doesn't matter what the man's profession is. You can have stronger testosterone release with even modest professions. An excellent barber will have more sustained T-spikes and trend lines than a doctor who is unsure of himself.

A client proudly told me, "I've been styling hair for twenty years, doctor, and I can do it with my eyes closed. Anything my customer wants, I can do. Crewcut, bowl cut, mushroom cut, Caesar cut, a flattop with a landing strip, spikey hair, Princeton cut, business man's cut, pompadour, French crop, wedge cut, whiffle cut, layer cut, feathered—you name it."

So master your job. Learn the new protocols, digital skills, manual skills, new processes, or the foreign language required. Update and upgrade yourself. Go to school part time, by correspondence, or on the Web. Go the extra distance to give yourself the competitive advantage against your peers. Then you can credibly chase a promotion you might be after. This sounds like sound business advice, but it's actually health advice based on testosterone chemistry.

An Immediate Sense of Reward or Accomplishment Enhances T

The brain decides constantly how much testosterone it will ask the testes to pour out. It's *that* dynamic, like a moment-to-moment vote, an instant approval rating, on your life.

Men who are paid for piecework, immediate fees for service, or commission have stronger testosterone rises than men on fixed salaries with no performance bonuses.

If you walk into a store, whether it's for men's clothing or electronics or fishing gear, you can immediately tell if the salespeople are on salary, or if they make commissions based on sales. Those who work on commissions have an active interest in making the sale, and will come after you. They will stalk you. Even if you just want to browse, or if you're being helped already, a salesperson will come and ask if you're being looked after.

The salaried salespeople may be just manning the store, and will get to you when they can. They are in no rush. You may have to search for one. Their lack of incentive leads to lack of initiative, which leads to dampened T-responses.

Incentives energize hormone spikes. T loves on-the-spot rewards.

So, set performance goals. Try to structure your work so that you can see the fruits of your own efforts directly. Arrange things as much as possible so that your work is performance based.

Even if that's not how you are compensated, you can still make a list of goals that you would like to achieve. Completing these tasks to your *own* satisfaction also caters to T-chemistry.

Working for Yourself

"I wish I had made the move years ago. As a software engineer, I used to service supply chain management clients for [one of the big computer manufacturers]. Six years ago, one of my colleagues and I decided to go out on our own and start our consultancy practice.

"I still remember when we got our first order . . . it was heaven. That order helped to cover our startup costs—all the servers, cooling systems, line time, backup generators, and redundant hardware.

"Now, we're sailing. We've got about sixty employees, just by sticking to our core competency. We now help buyers and suppliers interface globally . . . and it's all word of mouth. We don't even have to advertise anymore. I have enough that I don't have to work but I love to. . . . I should have made the move to be a consultant even earlier."

When you work for yourself, you control your own T-release to a much greater extent.

It's no secret that working for yourself is the best way to succeed. It's also the one common characteristic of wealthy people. You will have a special and deeper sense of reward—as long as you are successful, that is.

It also usually means that you are your own boss, competing only against other firms, or the market yourself, or against your own limitations. You don't have day-to-day disturbances from superiors coming down on you.

We know, for example, that a self-employed boss like our supply chain expert generally will have more forceful T-spikes than his employees.

ARM YOURSELF AGAINST CO-WORKERS WHO MAY DRAG YOU DOWN

> DO *NOT* MAKE a written list of irritating co-workers, which you keep at work.
>
> Clients have done this, and then their labeled list goes missing. . . .

Dealing with Co-Workers Who Irritate You

There are no special one-size-fits-all solutions for dealing with annoying co-workers. Dealing with such individuals will always be a work in progress. But it is important to understand that all organizations are full of politics and have people who bring you down. You should expect that a certain portion of your day will be negative. If you expect this, you will not be so surprised, annoyed, or bewildered when it happens. This protects your T.

Once you identify individuals in your work setting who may fall into these categories, you can be fully prepared. Essentially, it's a matter of shielding your T-levels from their negative assaults. Don't let them bring you or your hormone chemistry down.

Analyze your own workplace to see how many people fall into these classifications:

- The downer
- The credit thief
- The brown noser
- The backstabber
- The too important
- The user

> THERE ARE NO special solutions to these folks. But know that they exist in most organizations so you can protect yourself before encounters.

The Downer

"There's this assistant director in our branch, and I don't know why, but he always manages to make you feel bad after you've talked to him. He's a real downer. Either he will complain about the company, how he's being treated, how small his office his, how his parking spot is too far from the building, how he's the only one who knows what he's doing. . . . You wanna avoid him but you can't. He just makes you miserable."

Credit Thief

"I'm with an advertising agency based in New York and Los Angeles. One of our vice presidents, the bastard, always schedules client presentations when I'm on the other coast. He takes our group's ideas and presents them like they were all his own . . . he hogs the credit totally. If anything goes wrong, then of course it's our fault."

The Brown Noser

"One of our sales managers . . . I can't believe he pulled this one. At our company's annual meeting, we learned that our global CEO and some board members were going to stay on after the conference and go fly-fishing. So this guy schmoozes with the CEO at the opening-night cocktail reception and let's it drop that he's a fly-fishing expert, been a real enthusiast for years. So, of course, what does the CEO do? He invites him to join the group. . . . Now this guy didn't know the first thing about fly fishing. Nothing, *nada*. So the next three days he spends *learning how to fly-fish*. He even had videos and books couriered to him. And he pulled it off. Unbelievable."

Sucking up to one's superiors is a fine art in North American corporate life.

When you see one of your colleagues boot-licking, you feel a little destabilized. Your brain is thinking, "Should *I* be doing this, too? What if it works? Will it get me somewhere if I laugh at all the boss's jokes, or pretend that I'm really interested in his pursuits outside of work?"

The Backstabber

"I won an incentive trip. It was three days of meetings in Atlanta, plus a special executive retreat, expenses taken care of, the works. We were supposed to go alone, but my wedding anniversary was that weekend. I didn't want to miss the trip, I knew it would be good for my career, because all the top brass was going to be there.

"So I asked my wife to come along. I made sure I paid for her flight, but yes, obviously, she stayed with me in the same hotel room. Now the guy who I beat for this trip started this rumor that I expensed everything for my wife to the company. She never went to the hotel spa, but they're saying the company paid for all that too.

"And, you know, once the rumor is out, you can try to explain it away, but the damage is done. And the story gets worse with each telling as it circulates. . . . Next time, they'll be careful about giving me one of those trips, and you can be sure as hell that I won't be taking my wife with me then."

Another time-honored way to get ahead is by pulling other people down. Gossip, badmouthing, squealing, or just making up rumors is a traditional way to damage someone's reputation, good name, and future. Some people backstab by nature, others are more intelligent and choose their victim for maximum effect. They are more dangerous.

This type of direct attack will have direct hormonal effects: though bad-mouthing doesn't draw blood, it does draw testosterone.

> THE VICTIM OF a backstabber will see his T diminish.
> On the other hand, the person doing the backstabbing will see his T rise. And the better he thinks he's nailing his intended victim, the more his T rises. (This is not an endorsement of backstabbing, just an explanation of its realities.)
> *Why* does a man's T rise when he's badmouthing a co-worker? This seems to be part of the predator in us, the kill-or-be-killed instinct. Our T rises if we make someone else's T fall.

The Too Important

"We were at a management meeting. All the senior decision makers were there. So this one colleague, you can just see how she works the room. Like a magnet, she goes straight to all the managers. She chats them all up, with her *oh-so-pleasant* three-minute routine with each of them.

"She won't even bother to say hello to anyone else, even if she's right in front of you. And you think to yourself, you know, our jobs are comparable. I'm not a junior employee. But she only zones in on people who can help her get ahead.... It is so obvious and annoying, and it happens like clockwork."

Too-self-important individuals may not be overtly negative to you. They just see themselves as floating in a higher orbit. They think that your position or power can't benefit them in any way. So they don't even extend simple courtesies to you.

> THIS COUSIN OF brown-nosing tends to be a mild irritant but happens recurrently. It's also a reminder that you may not be at the top of the pecking order (yet).

The User

"There's a colleague of mine at work, and I like him. But, you know, after a while it gets a bit annoying. He's always asking me to do some invoicing and cross-checking for him. I made the mistake of offering to do it once, now he just asks me to do it too much.... I still do it. He's polite, we discuss office matters. But now I know his game.

"He'll come over to me, a few minutes of general conversation, and then casually ask me for this favor... shamelessly. It's ridiculous. Every time without fail.... But, that's it. No more. It's not my job to do this for him anyway. I know he'll be offended, probably won't speak to me, but I have responsibilities too."

There will be people at work who are friendly to you but have ulterior motives. Fairly quickly, you realize that the only reason they are so pleasant is so that you can get something done for them.

One signal of this is that the only time they really talk to you is when they need something. There's little, if any, social chit-chat in between requests, little interest in you or your needs. If they don't need anything, they don't talk.

Recognize Which of Your Work Colleagues Fit These Classifications

Learn in advance to identify the people who can bring you down, so you can prepare your mind, your responses, for the inevitable encounters. This way, you can be on alert, strategize, put up deflector shields, let annoyances bounce off you, and preserve your testosterone integrity.

Do not let such people talk to you without your being on guard, as it can take a while to purge yourself of the encounter.

Do not waste time, energy, and testosterone by holding silent grudges, reliving conversations, or thinking up what you *should* have said to tell them off, after the fact. If you do this you are brooding, and burning off your T for no reason.

> IN NORTH AMERICA, having to deal with annoying or ungrateful co-workers or work groups is one of the chief reasons for leaving a job.

Dealing with Your Boss

"I screwed up big. We lost a major advertising client to one of our rival firms. My boss called me in to see him, and walking to his office was the longest walk of my life. . . . I thought he was going to fire me on the spot, but he didn't.

"He told me that he knew my area of focus and specialization was consumer products, so I had no business being in with the pharmaceutical marketing group. He said he still thinks I do valuable work, but I've got to be more careful, because the pharma guys aren't as free-wheeling as consumer brand managers.

"He also told me that I shouldn't be learning a new product focus on a major account. He goes, 'That's not the time for training wheels.' What I did might have jeopardized our accounts with other brand managers in the same drug company, their other in-house products.

"I was pretty relieved. Sure, I thought, 'Great, five years of my life down the drain over one client. . . . ' Sometimes we think we can do it all. But there's a skill to everything, and you shouldn't bite off more than you can chew. I'm grateful to be able to prove myself again."

Your boss can make or break your testosterone.

When you're in the same room with your boss, your T is more fragile, and the spikes are larger, either up or down, depending on whether it's a positive or negative encounter.

Because of his or her position of power over you, your boss has a particular ability to amplify up or bleed down your T trend lines. An encounter with your boss can affect your T-disposition from hours to days, especially if you receive a dressing-down, a talking-to, disciplinary action, or a bad performance review.

This is part of the feeling of nervousness when you're in the presence of authority, in the presence of the person who signs your checks, could fire you if you don't walk the line, and could set you back years if he or she wanted to.

It is important to cultivate a mutually respectful relationship with your boss. Let your boss learn about your competencies, your drive and energy, and your special skills. Show your employer that you are serious about your work, and not just time-serving or clock-watching. Get passionate about your work and let him or her see that. This buys a little credit, as well as T-protection, if anything unfavorable happens to you in the future.

MAKE SURE YOU BOND WITH YOUR LOVED ONE(S) *DAILY*

"Daddy, when I grow up, can I be your client, too, so we can have a meeting?"

Many men give so much of themselves to their work that they exclude family and their loved one(s). They travel too much, spend excess time at meetings, work overtime to make the big bucks, take extra shifts, and take on too much responsibility. Men are always explaining away their absence, that they need time to work, and protest that they will definitely spend more time with their family later. This "later" never comes.

Neglecting loved ones is a grave mistake—not only for the family, but also for the man's own health.

> WHEN WE FLOAT our egos on the open market, and look to that rough arena to prop us up, to give us our T-boosts, we live at the world's whim.
>
> That's dangerous, and that's why we need anchoring, ego-building personal relationships.

Feeling loved, wanted, and needed, not for your title or job skills or power or earning capacity—*just for being you*—is a mighty testosterone builder. Warm relationships are an antidote to the testosterone circus of work life.

"Soft time" with family is necessary for grounding, for orientation, for keeping you whole and moored, and for keeping you stable and real.

> ### Sports and Male Psychological Health
>
> WHEN MEN GET their T smashed at work, they will often turn to watching pro sports as a substitute source of T-enrichment.
>
> One wife asks, "What is it with men and all these sports, these teams? Is it that important that Boston beats Chicago, or that Los Angeles beats Miami? Who cares? . . . I think men should calm down and grow up."
>
> Of course, playing sports is better than watching them. But even watching them, being a committed fan, influences hormones, especially when it's playoff time.
>
> Cheering for their team, taking an active interest, going to games to feel the roar of the crowd in the stadium, watching matches on TV, taking it personally—all these build their testosterone supply.
>
> How their team does can be a personal matter of honor for many men. When *real* fans watch their team win, their testosterone

surges. The more important the game, the greater the T-rise, and the longer the aftereffects. Similarly, when real fans watch their favorite athletes lose, especially during the run-up to the pennant, playoffs, or championship, it depresses their testosterone.

This is the biochemical importance of major-league sports, and one of the reasons that men take these games so seriously. But men should also try to spend bonding time with their family as their source of T-renewal. This is deeper and longer lasting than investing so much emotion in a game.

"My own dad worked a lot of overtime when I was a kid. He himself was a young father and wanted to do his best to support his family. Despite this, my dad was always a big part of my life because when he *was* home, he made me a priority. He made the time we had together quality 'father-son' time.

"This is really important for me now with my own kids. It's not easy, but I do try to give them the quality time that they deserve. . . . I think quality is better than quantity."

The important lesson in all this is, the next time you have trouble or a challenge at work, you need support outside of work to get you through it. Your family will be the ones who will be there for you in these situations.

The definition of family is broad, too. It may be your father or mother that you retreat to in times of stress, or own brother or sister, or the wife and kids, or a life partner. Whatever your primary group or your primary source of affection, build it, cultivate it, make sure it's not rusty, make sure it's still in working order.

The downtime you spend with a loving family or social support is the sanctuary time to rebuild testosterone strength. It's like intensive care delivered at home.

16

Relationships

A MEMBER OF the First Wives' Club, a forty-six-year-old woman, is one of my favorite clients. I enjoy her frank and open conversation, which has a dark and biting humor. She was divorced last year after three kids, two dogs, two renovations, and fifteen years of marriage. "Hey, doc, have you heard about the three kinds of sex?" she asked me in my clinic.

"No, I haven't," I replied with a smile. I could see the mischief in her face.

"There's three kinds of sex: house sex, bedroom sex, and hallway sex. House sex is when you're just married. Everything's hot and bothered. You have sex in every room of the house, in the bathtub, in the kitchen, on the dining table, kind of like inaugurating each room.

"After a while you settle down into a routine. The passion kind of goes, you know what to expect, it's a habit, so you only have sex in the bedroom.

"Hallway sex happens after many years. By then, you're barely speaking to each other. So when you pass each other in the hallway, you just say, 'Fuck you.'"

LOVE CHANGES EVERYTHING, including testosterone.

How does a man's testosterone chemistry relate to his relationships? While there are no magic solutions to the riddle of relationships, learning how your hormone chemistry is affected by your partner can help.

Learning about T-chemistry will allow you to better understand your own psyche, buried emotions, hidden motivations, chemical reward systems, brain triggers, and behavior patterns. Even those men with good, low scores in the following questionnaire could benefit from the information and exercises in this chapter.

You will also learn to recognize and resist some of the negative tendencies that T can lead to over time.

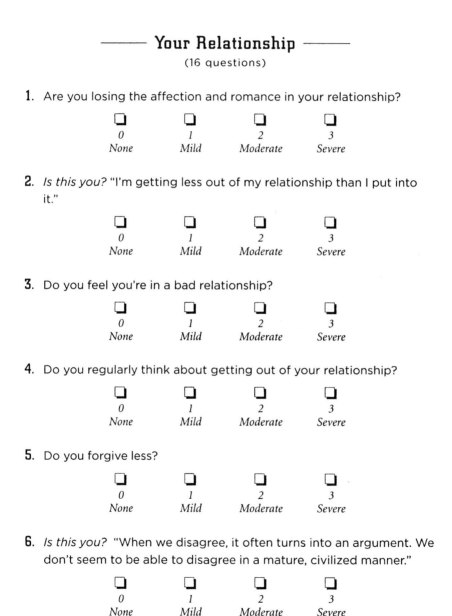

———— Your Relationship ————
(16 questions)

1. Are you losing the affection and romance in your relationship?

☐	☐	☐	☐
0	*1*	*2*	*3*
None	*Mild*	*Moderate*	*Severe*

2. *Is this you?* "I'm getting less out of my relationship than I put into it."

☐	☐	☐	☐
0	*1*	*2*	*3*
None	*Mild*	*Moderate*	*Severe*

3. Do you feel you're in a bad relationship?

☐	☐	☐	☐
0	*1*	*2*	*3*
None	*Mild*	*Moderate*	*Severe*

4. Do you regularly think about getting out of your relationship?

☐	☐	☐	☐
0	*1*	*2*	*3*
None	*Mild*	*Moderate*	*Severe*

5. Do you forgive less?

☐	☐	☐	☐
0	*1*	*2*	*3*
None	*Mild*	*Moderate*	*Severe*

6. *Is this you?* "When we disagree, it often turns into an argument. We don't seem to be able to disagree in a mature, civilized manner."

☐	☐	☐	☐
0	*1*	*2*	*3*
None	*Mild*	*Moderate*	*Severe*

7. *Is this you?* "We argue too frequently."

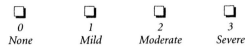

   0   1   2   3
 None   Mild   Moderate   Severe

8. When you argue, do you explode like a volcano, hurling insults at your partner?

   0   1   2   3
 None   Mild   Moderate   Severe

9. *Is this you?* "When my kids were young, they slept in our bed, right up until they were about five or six years old."

   0   1   2   3
 None   Mild   Moderate   Severe

10. If you have a fight, can a lot of time go by without speaking to each other—because of a domestic cold war?

   0   1   2   3
 None   Mild   Moderate   Severe

11. Do you think about having an affair, and wish you had the guts to have one?

   0   1   2   3
 None   Mild   Moderate   Severe

12. *Is this you?* "I am ready to *receive* affection, but I don't give it so much."

   0   1   2   3
 None   Mild   Moderate   Severe

13. Does your partner feel you're married to your computer?

   0   1   2   3
 None   Mild   Moderate   Severe

14. *Is this you?* "I don't know why, but I remember my old girlfriends more, even the ones who got away. They'll just pop into my mind—memories of some of my encounters from earlier days."

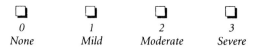

0	1	2	3
None	*Mild*	*Moderate*	*Severe*

15. *Is this you?* "I don't get the support I need from my partner. I'll suggest some idea or scheme, and I'll get one of those *here-we-go-again* looks."

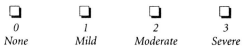

0	1	2	3
None	*Mild*	*Moderate*	*Severe*

16. *Is this you?* Your partner wants *to talk,* and asks how your day was. You're thinking, "Oh God, give it a rest, will you? Just leave me alone." You give brush-off replies, "Fine, yeah, everything's fine. Nothing's wrong."

0	1	2	3
None	*Mild*	*Moderate*	*Severe*

Your Relationship

Your score:_____/ 48 points

Score/Rating

0 to 5	*None*
6 to 19	*Mild*
20 to 38	*Moderate*
39 to 48	*Severe*

Consider your score range here—is it None, Mild, Moderate, or Severe? Your score will help you determine how urgently you need the recommendations in this chapter.

Key Points
- Intimate relationships change your testosterone dynamics.
- Your changing need for testosterone will change your relationship.
- After age forty, you will begin to feel the changes, and your body and behavior will start to shift.

The underlying premise:

A man's body wants its testosterone hits. Parts of long-term relationships cater to this, parts block this. This dynamic struggle continues all the time.

The struggle becomes more important once a man is over forty.

In midlife, a man may not feel he is getting the T-boost that he's used to. Other areas of his life may not be offering the same hormonal enrichment as before—because of his own fading health, poor sleep, poor diet, routine sex, excess stress, job strain, and so on.

His body seeks T, and his behavior and personality slowly shift to *get* that T. His relationship may suffer.

WHAT TO DO

- Learn what you're up against—the background numbers of long-term relationships.
- Be aware of how testosterone changes your relationship and personality over the years of being together.
- Move towards a more successful relationship.

LEARN WHAT YOU'RE UP AGAINST—THE BACKGROUND NUMBERS OF RELATIONSHIPS

What makes a successful relationship? It seems nobody knows for sure. Certainly, relationship counselors don't know. It's bizarre, but relationship counselors themselves break up about 5 to 10 percent more than the general population.

Counseling can have benefits, but what's not appreciated is the hand of physiology, the percolating hormones under the surface. Despite the billions of dollars spent by North Americans on relationship therapy, the end results—was your relationship saved, improved, or made happier?—generally aren't any different than if you went at it on your own. That's because the push and pull of hormones are not recognized by therapists who focus on just the social dynamics of a relationship. But that can change once you understand the nature of testosterone.

It's time to empower couples with advice based on the biology of testosterone chemistry.

> **A MAN DIES four to seven years earlier if he's not in a long-term relationship.**
>
> It's *not* from starvation, as some women have sarcastically suggested—that no one is there to cook for him.

> One of the real reasons for this lowered life expectancy is that the single man is not receiving the T-hits and care that a good relationship can provide.

Relationships Are Fragile

More than half of all relationships end in separation. Many relationships break up in the first two years. At that early stage, people may realize they are incompatible, or that they were in lust and not love, or that their personalities clash too much.

But another separation point is in midlife, usually after ten to fifteen years of union. This is shocking.

You'd think that partners who had spent that much time together would have figured things out, would understand each other, and cut each other some slack. You'd think they would have gone through enough arguments to having a working cease-fire.

So the question arises—what changes in the relationship lead to a break-up?

Are You Drifting Apart?

Do you go to bed at separate times?

Generally this means you're living separate lives, and is a marker for couples who drift apart.

Are You Cheating?

About 23 million North American men have been unfaithful to their spouses. The illicit sex may be good for their testosterone, but it's bad for their domestic relationship.

Sex in an affair burns up to five times as many calories as sex with your routine partner.

That's partly why when you cheat, you experience such a T-burst, which can be two to four times greater than occurs with your routine partner.

The body senses this, somehow knowing it without having to do the scientific measurements. This is not an endorsement of cheating, but a discussion of the chemistry.

BE AWARE OF HOW TESTOSTERONE CHANGES YOUR RELATIONSHIP AND PERSONALITY OVER THE YEARS OF BEING TOGETHER

The Chase Is More Thrilling than The Capture

Testosterone spikes during the thrill of a chase, challenge, the courting, and the uncertainty of the early days of the relationship.

Once you are in a stable relationship, the novelty wears off, and this blunts your T-spikes.

After about one or two years, a couple will become so familiar, so used to each other, that the man will no longer receive the same T-enrichment as before.

Part of a Man's Difficulty in Committing to a Relationship is Testosterone Based

To commit to a long-term relationship, a man's body unconsciously has to say, "I choose *you* and give you the major responsibility to be there for my testosterone needs, to the exclusion of all others, for the rest of my days."

That can be a challenge. Even while the excitement and attraction are at their peak, the conscious anticipation of falling into a more routine relationship has an effect on testosterone

As a result, men who are about to enter into a long-term relationship have wild T-swings, with rapid rises and falls. This is one of the reasons men can be so jittery before making a romantic commitment.

After the Honeymoon Period, Testosterone Decreases

People who enter into stable relationships very early in life, let's say in their first relationship, whether this involves marriage or not, tend not to stay together. Part of that breakup is because both partners may have been immature, not ready for the commitment, and so on.

But another part of the reason is that a man's T declines after the honeymoon period. The earlier he does this in life, the more his body will rebel.

His body unconsciously thinks, "Why did I give up all those possible partners, and all the T-rushes that were still coming to me? Is this all there is?"

The Midlife Testosterone Slump

Men over forty experience testosterone withdrawal. That's what it resembles medically. Consider an analogy to oxygen:

Oxygen is absolutely essential, allowing us to burn energy. Without it, our brains die within six minutes.

We all inhale about sixteen to twenty times per minute, breathing in oxygen from the outside air. The amount of oxygen in our bloodstream is strictly guarded and calibrated. At any time, within seconds, if our onboard chemical detectors in the brain, like a built-in smoke alarm, sense that we need more oxygen, many things can happen. Maybe it's something simple— perhaps we yawn, taking in extra air, restoring the balance. This just happens; it's all done internally, and you're not really part of the decision. The yawning mechanism is part of the automatic (autonomic) nervous system. You can try to stop the yawn, mask it, hide it for polite society—but the body will be satisfied, it *will* have its yawn.

If the body really needs oxygen, then we might panic, run to fresher air, reach for an emergency oxygen mask, faint, or worse. This all happens quickly, dramatically, and in plain view.

Testosterone is like oxygen. It's too important for the body to give up easily. It's what the man's body is used to. T is essential for many feelings, abilities, and keeping the body tuned, revved, and energetic. A man's body does not appreciate losing this manhood chemical, so it reacts. The body will change gears, fight, go after new interests, pursuits, partners, or sexual experiences to restore this necessary chemical balance.

And the body *will* be satisfied. It will maintain its hormone supply, and the excitements that we go after release T from our onboard pharmacy. Instructions are issued from deep within, well below our awareness, and these are what lead to the personality, physical, and emotional changes we do notice. In the case of both T and oxygen, our onboard brain detectors rule.

The difference is in the timing: the decline in oxygen happens over seconds, and the body's remedies do, too. The decline in T happens over years, and the body's remedies do, too.

Shifts in a Man's Personality Tend to Begin at about Age Forty

The midlife man's T-production may be blunted by lifestyle choices, such as poor eating, excess stress, weight gain, and so on. So his body will start to go after its hormonal rush in other ways.

CLASSIC SELF-PRESCRIPTION: **The old treatments for midlife challenges:**
- A new hairstyle
- A new sports car
- A new relationship

And the modern addition of:
- Plastic surgery for a new chin, nose, wrinkle-free face, or liposuctioned abdomen.

The one element common to these approaches is that they all lead to T-enrichment. They are T-rescues.

A man's body craves and seeks testosterone enrichment. He will get that T through either positive or negative actions—and his body *doesn't care* which.

These are some positive actions that lead to T-boosts:

- Valuing your relationship because you think your partner is wonderful

- Feeling loved and valued
- Being told you are special
- Anticipating serious sex
- Being proud of your partner, showing him or her off
- Getting your ego puffed up
- Feeling excited by shopping for electronics, software, stereo equipment, and the latest sports gear
- Showing off your luxury gadgets

These are all actions to be encouraged, even if your partner may consider some of them foolish. At worst, they are harmless, at best beneficial. Because, consider this—a man will also get a hormonal boost by other, not-so-desirable actions. These are negative actions that *also* lead to T-boosts:

- Flirting with an attractive co-worker
- Swearing in anger, reasserting your position
- Arguing strongly to overcome an insult
- Acting out a jealous rage
- Road rage as a way of scaring the passenger
- Feeling clever because you got away with deceit
- Successfully taking revenge
- Having an affair
- Planning or imagining breaking up with a partner, and looking forward to having freedom to play the field

These are actions that lead to T-declines:

- Feeling neglected and being taken for granted
- Being told you are awful
- Being denied sex
- Feeling that you disappoint your partner
- Getting your ego smashed down
- Being asked to admit mistakes and to make a sincere apology
- Losing an argument
- Being ridiculed and laughed at
- Getting sworn at in anger
- Feeling stupid because you got caught doing something
- Arguing with your in-laws
- Discovering more and more that your partner is not as wonderful as you thought
- Feeling that you're trapped in your relationship, that you have lost your freedom to play the field

---

Partners as Teachers

IT IS ESPECIALLY important for partners to understand what their midlife men may go through.

By knowing about T-chemistry, both women and men can better anticipate, prepare for, endure, and overcome the hormonally driven changes in their man's behavior and personality.

A special note to women: Women are usually the ones who teach men about health and well-being issues. Once the women understand a problem that concerns the body, then they can teach their men to deal with it—because the men themselves just don't seem to take their own health seriously.

In a long-term relationship, a man may attempt to rebalance and recapture his reduced T by using negative approaches.

As men enter their midlife, they receive fewer positive T-enrichments. They encounter more hormone-diminishing actions. And they get more and more hormonal enrichment through negative actions.

This strains relationships during midlife, and is part of the reason for the significant numbers of breakups at this life stage. In fact, about 25 percent of all long-term commitments end in midlife.

You *can* override your testosterone hunger with your conscious will. But the push, the tendency to seek T, to act in negative ways to get or boost it, is always there, always lurking under the hood.

At Midlife, Men Become More Easily Irritated

As men enter their forties, they develop a shorter fuse, stay angry longer, and tend to blow up more easily.

This phenomenon now even has its own name—the irritable male syndrome.

Unfortunately, an expression of anger and irritability and guarding of their territory—all these things increase T.

This becomes more common after age forty. It can happen like the flip of a switch.

Recall that T-production is monitored constantly and reacts in real time to what's going on. This turning on and off of a temper, of accusations, bewilders and may even frighten partners.

Many partners begin to wonder just who it is they've been with for so long. To varying degrees, this midlife hormonal shift changes a man's personality. That's why so many partners thought that they knew everything about their man but are then surprised to see these changes.

A wife of nineteen years said, "I am thirty-nine now, and my husband is forty-five. Sometimes I think he's got two personalities, a real Jekyll and Hyde split. One minute, he'll be all jokey and kind, and the next minute he'll explode. Maybe he didn't like what I said or something, but the way he boils over is *too* much. . . . I'm scared that I'll say the wrong thing and set him off."

Is Your Partner a Blame Magnet?

DO YOU FEEL that everything is your partner's fault? Are you easily annoyed and irritated by your partner? Do you consider most of your partner's conversation nagging? Midlife men can have tempers that boil over remarkably easily, way beyond even their usual emotions.

The Temptation to Play Around

The husband says: "Sure, I love Roberta . . . I never stopped loving her. But I couldn't tell her that she didn't turn me on enough anymore. This was building for years, and I missed it. I started noticing other women more. I mean I'd always been faithful up till then. I really wasn't looking to have an affair. Maybe I was just born to be wild."

What he says about the redhead, his new love interest: "I'm not a bad person, honestly. I felt a need. She made me feel like a knight in shining armor. She made me feel important, she loved my hands. I felt like a man, like I could do no wrong. She even said she missed the sound of my voice. C'mon, when was the last time Roberta said that to me? Probably before we were married."

The chemical explanation of the husband's behavior: Certainly, the husband made a choice to stray, redhead or no redhead. His body was used to having a good supply of testosterone, and this had been declining for several years as the midlife challenges set in.

His body had been issuing orders from within, below his level of awareness, which he had resisted for years. Now, having an affair, fresh sexual experiences, being admired and valued, dressing to be noticed, and not being taken for granted—all these behaviors boosted his ego. This in turn gave him the T-rush, the chemical burst, that his body and his sense of manhood craved.

This is not a justification or invitation for having affairs, but an explanation of the chemistry involved. Another, flip-side, set of midlife feelings relates to this:

The Chemistry of Jealousy

If a man believes his partner is flirting with another man, it causes an immediate and intense downward spike in his own testosterone (and, by the way, the T of the person *doing* the flirting increases). The man, momentarily T-deprived, can erupt. A jealous rage reasserts the testosterone level by reaffirming his turf and territory. His body is declaring, in its own primitive way, "That's my partner, don't come near."

One client remembered her husband's jealousy: "We were at an office Christmas party, and I was talking to his colleagues. *His* colleagues, you understand? I went because Nathaniel [her husband] wanted us to go. . . . I talked to one guy, he was an executive vice president, for a few minutes. We were just being sociable. But later, when we were leaving, Nate just blew up, right there in the parking lot. We didn't even make it to the car. He was so jealous. As if I'd done God-knows-what. He accused me of . . . well, let's say he said some pretty awful things."

Whether it was true or not, her husband felt that she was being enticed by another man, he felt challenged, and his brain sensed an imminent threat. He could have overridden this inner reaction, he could have reasoned his way through it, shown a little civilized behavior, but he didn't.

The most extreme version of this reaction occurs in a man who will not accept that a relationship is ending or over. Twenty-five percent of all physical injuries to women that occur in the workplace are caused by current, estranged, or former partners.

> **IT SHOULD COME** as no surprise that even destructive actions can raise testosterone levels.
>
> **High-octane, high-T activities are not always uplifting, pleasant, or catering to the greater good.**

This jealous rage is part of our heritage from our evolutionary past, part of the behaviors of early man.[1] If a man sees his partner being approached, courted, touched, or flirted with by another male, it's a threat to his dominance, to his place in society, to his place in the pride. It's an assault on his manhood, a threat to his masculinity.

Like the emergency need for oxygen, the body demands action. The body will be satisfied. It *will* maintain its T-supply.

---

[1]We must admit we are somewhat suspicious of evolutionary explanations of current behavior that tie us to a distant past. Are we only cavemen temporarily and tentatively civilized? Naked apes? One would hope that we've progressed beyond the basic, gritty instincts of early man, and broken out of those constraints. But perhaps we only dress better. (This explanation of the value of a jealous rage, that it raises T, the manhood chemical, is the best one so far, but we're hopeful a more complimentary reason will be found in the future.)

The "Value" of a Jealous Rage

A jealous rage restores T. Whether the man confronts the offending male or his own partner, the expression of jealousy reasserts his manhood, reaffirms his status in his own mind, and preserves the pecking order, thereby resulting in an upward spike of T.

Interestingly, to restore T levels, you can't just *feel* jealous. It can't be a passive, disappointed brooding, as that does not change testosterone levels much. You can't just be a spectator.

To raise the level of the manhood chemical, it has to be an active jealous rage, acted out with enthusiasm, preferably with invigorating shouting and shaking of fists. That will do the job. (This is *not* to condone violent behavior, but it does illustrate what the body itself demands, and how body chemistry plays its role.)

But even better, try to work with your partner toward more T-enhancing activities you may achieve in harmony.

MOVE TOWARD A SUCCESSFUL RELATIONSHIP

One of the problems we notice in busy, midlife couples is that they're often living like roommates. They just check in with each other, make sure the fridge is stocked, have routine sex lives, and are just too busy to experience the softer moments of life. This is one of the major sources of T-renewal that gets pushed to the side in the modern world, and we need as a society to allow ourselves these moments to reconnect.

Many observations can be made about successful relationships. The recommendations in this section come from my two decades of dealing with thousands of midlife men. These actions will either directly elevate your T-levels, indirectly help you avoid T-crashes, or buy you some credit. They are not mere generalizations but are related to T-chemistry.

Let Your Past Relationships Remain Forgotten

T-crash:

> *Your spouse picks up a book in your home, and out falls a lovely photo of you with your arm around an ex-girlfriend. This scenario usually demands a lot of jittery apologizing and explaining away. Meanwhile, your T plummets.*

If your current partner angrily confronts you about a past relationship—even though it's *in the past*—men often feel guilty, caught out, almost as if they had been unfaithful. This smashes your T-levels, and is actually an efficient way of demoralizing you.

When men commit to a long-term relationship, they like to come clean, revealing all their past relationships and entanglements.

Do not do this.

Whatever you disclose will come back to haunt you, I promise.

What you reveal in unguarded moments of sincerity may become ammunition during an argument, or in some other context. It doesn't always happen, but enough men have suffered because of disclosures about their own past that I think it's important to mention.

For example, when a man commits to a long-term relationship, he often has to clean house and get rid of old photos, letters, books, papers, and mementos—all the reminders of past relationships. As you dump all those items, let the memories and mention of them also disappear.

Don't Have the Same Argument Again and Again

Couples argue about the same issues for years. They are caught in a loop that drains their energies.

Topics include:

- Your mother is too involved in our lives.
- Why don't you give up these crazy diets?
- Why can't you ever answer the phone?
- Who do you think you are, lord of the manor?
- How many pairs of shoes can you buy?
- Why are you such a shopaholic?
- Can't you try to be nice to my family?
- Why are we supposed to be responsible for your family's business problems?
- Can't you see that we can't afford that right now?
- Why do you always spoil my new projects?
- Why can't you discipline the kids properly?
- Do we have to buy that just because our neighbors did?
- Why can't you fix the things around the house faster?
- Is watching that game really that important?

And so on.

If you find yourself arguing about approximately the same issues, resolve this. It's not easy to achieve, but you must move beyond this kind of constant complaining and bickering.

Seek counseling if you have to. Have a summit conference, deal with these recurring, festering problems, and don't let them gather more venom.

Arguments that are allowed to recur over years eventually become toxic and radioactive, leaving a trail of destruction. It's precisely these perpetual arguments, these unresolved, always-in-the-air disagreements that push your buttons, that lead to T-diminishment.

Spend Time with Each Other That Is Not Goal Oriented, Enjoying Each Other's Conversation—No Sex Here

Give yourselves time to reconnect as companions.

What Does Your Mate Feel Like?

A workplace widow?
A golf widow?
An Internet widow?
A television widow?
An I'm-out-with-the-guys-tonight widow?

Do you feel as if everything else in her life is more important than you—the kids, her responsibilities, her friends, her family, her job?

Couples are overstretched—running a household, dealing with endless responsibilities, and making ends meet. We often see partners consumed by their workaday lives, or by interests they do not share. It seems quite simple, but couples forget to have unpressured, free-floating fun together.

Slow down occasionally, have protected, exclusive time together—say, every two to three weeks or so.

Block out unstructured time to be alone together regularly—when you don't have to pay any bills, answer phone calls, shop for groceries, drive kids to events, get things repaired, pick up dry cleaning, keep appointments, attend meetings, and so on.

In this way, you are reconnecting with your partner, and giving her protected time to rev up your T-chemistry. If you do not do this, you will drift even further apart.

Try to Communicate

Testosterone seems to build a shield around the man's inner personality.

Communicating with your partner, when *she* asks for it and you don't feel like it, can actually reduce your testosterone. You feel threatened or irritated.

But communicating when *you* want to actually raises your testosterone.

There is a book with a great title, which says it all: *If Men Could Talk.* Or to play on a movie title, *Look Who's (Not) Talking.*

If you do not regularly communicate with your partner, negative emotions will stockpile over the years, and these will simmer and brew internally. This will be toxic to both partners, and to your testosterone.

Communicating is easier said than done, because testosterone actually seems to build a cocoon around a man's core personality.

It seems that men, for at least part of the day, ideally want to be valued and admired in cold heroic silence. Generally not wanting to talk about emotional problems, finding it hard to apologize, men often don't even realize that they've done anything wrong. All of these things together infuriate their partners, and damage relationships.

Typical questions may be asked in complete conversational innocence by the partner:

- "So, how was your day?"
- "What happened at work?"
- "What are you thinking?"
- "Anything important happen?"

But testosterone chemistry reveals that men feel differently when asked these questions. Their T-levels diminish, because men think they are being scrutinized and inspected. Men seem to think they're being interviewed, assessed, even audited. To them, it is not simply a private, nonthreatening conversation with a loved one, but an unwarranted interrogation.

It's fascinating, but men feel as if their partner is prying, as if she wants to know some private information that the man doesn't want to divulge, or couldn't be bothered to share.

So you should try to overcome this tendency towards silence, avoiding emotions, or turning inward into a cocoon, as this can chronically offend your partner.

Does This Conversation Sound Familiar?

"So, how was your day?" she asks.

"Hmmm," he replies.

"Sweetie, I'm *asking* you how your day was."

"Hmmm. Good," he replies.

"Is that your answer?" she persists.

"Yes, my day was fine. All right?"

"Anything important happen?" she wants to know.

"No, everything's fine, *okay*," he concludes this interaction, with slightly raised voice.

Part of the explanation for the legendary, short, brush-off

answers that men give to these questions when they're vegging out in front of the television in the evening is related to T-chemistry. Inexplicably, men may feel as if they're being audited, even inspected, when asked these innocent questions. This downspikes their T, and they give curt replies.

Date Each Other Even after You've Been in a Long-Term Relationship

Give yourselves time and opportunities to reconnect. Date each other regularly, although it is difficult with all the responsibilities couples set for themselves.

Suggestions include: dinner at a fancy restaurant, weekend getaways, at-home bubble baths (not with water that's too hot), picnics, a day at the spa for two, and gallery walks. This is all about breaking your set patterns, your routine, and rekindling your relationship.

Learn to Flirt with Each Other Again

Show some affection in public. Scandalize your kids. Put your arm around your partner. Hold hands when you walk. French-kiss on the way out to work once in a while. Stroke your partner's behind or knee secretly, or play footsie, when other people are nearby. Touch each other even—especially—when you can't consummate what you start.

Rekindle the excitement in significant glances at each other across a room, in using a privately sexual language in front of other people who won't catch the secret. Whisper in her ear once in a while.

Something about this being illicit, that you might be caught, actually builds testosterone and heightens the pleasure of the whole experience.

Be Sensual

When was the last time you brushed her hair, or shampooed it for her? Give her a full-body massage.

These small, unexpected moments of affection and caring can go a long way to rebond, and this caters to T over time by (re)building intimacy and trust.

Cuddle Without Sex

"He never kisses me, or shows any affection unless he wants sex. Sometimes I just want affection, and don't want intercourse every time. Why can't he learn to be tender?"

On occasion, cuddle your partner to show affection, not as a prelude to sex. (Re)learn how to be comfortably close. For example, when you watch a movie together at home, sit behind your partner and hold her in your arms for the duration of the film.

Have a Vigorous Sex Life

> THAT'S WHY THEY call it *sexual healing.*

"We're so busy that I'm having sex about once every two weeks."

You need time, you need energy, you need some degree of relaxation, and preferably not on too tight a schedule, to have good sex.

Take showers together.

There are all kinds of ways to demonstrate that you're still a man, still virile. It doesn't always have to be penetrating intercourse.

Do other things. Learn about the many definitions of sex. Expand your concept of foreplay. Experience this (re)awakening together.

See the Sex chapter.

Have a Positive Sense of Humor

One of the few things in this world that you cannot rent is a sense of humor. If you've misplaced yours, find it.

Note: the humor is supposed to be positive, not mean-spirited. That means you're to laugh about other things, outside things, the world, your predicament, your day, your neighbor. Not about each other.

Do not mock each other, or tear down what a partner cares about.

Unfortunately, you *will* actually get a testosterone spike if you have a negative, sarcastic, insulting kind of humor. Basically, you are building yourself up by diminishing your partner.

This is why this teasing, biting, critical humor is so common between couples. It's certainly not very pleasant, and it causes ego-strain on your partner too. And no doubt your partner will come back at you, and the cycle will continue.

> *MOCKING EACH OTHER?* "My wife is always laughing or making fun of my gray hair. Okay, I've earned it. With all the stuff I've gone through and put up with, who wouldn't have gray hair by now? I'm not interested in coloring my gray: I like it. If she's got a problem with it, well, we'll just have to figure that out."

Learn to Apologize, or to Let Some Arguments End in a Draw

Apologizing is an admission of error, a seeking of forgiveness, a guilty plea. To do this, a man has to willfully orchestrate his own testosterone decline. Not an easy feat.

For a man to apologize seems to be a biochemical challenge. He can do it, but his conscious will has to override his chemical tendencies.

At the very least, you don't have to win every argument, you don't have to take a stand, you don't have to let your views always be clearly and loudly and forcefully known. Mellow out a bit and let things go. Recognize that letting go is counter to your hormonal impulse, contrary to the upsurge of chemicals triggered by conflict.

Many couples recall that it was during the heat of an argument that they said their final words. The desire to win the argument is what leads to behavior and words that are out of control, and is particularly destructive.

Alcohol and Arguments

DO NOT ADD alcohol to an argument. Alcohol leads to uncontrolled behavior, domestic violence, even femicide.

Do Not Call Your Partner Names

Ex-wife: "I have no respect left for him. I don't think I'm a bitch at all, but he pushes my buttons. Maybe he turns me into one. . . . I'm not putting up with it anymore."

Again, this sounds basic, simple, and self-evident. But names are what get remembered. They're what get replayed back to you, what your partner's friends will be told, what children will repeat, what extended family will learn, and possibly a lawyer, too. It's names that linger and damage and resurface.

Your own words may be used against you by well-informed lawyers, proving how hostile and hurtful you were.

Purge insulting words from your vocabulary, particularly your anger vocabulary.

Anger-words show deep contempt, are hard to take back, are really difficult to apologize for, and can even affect custody battles.

Be warned.

Exit Strategy

It had to end: "I think we were in love, at least at the beginning. But it's so many arguments ago. I'm not really sure where the bitterness came from. Sure, his family interfered in our lives, and when we moved to our neighborhood, he spent too much time with his drinking buddies. Poker, beer, baseball, hockey— whatever. He always had time for everyone else except us. . . . What can I say? We tried, but twelve years later it's over. It's painful for me to say this—I can't believe these words are coming out of me—but it's best to move on."

When I started my practice a couple of decades ago, doctors in my field were always thinking of our work as being heroic. We thought that all marriages could and should be saved. But we have learned that sometimes people really are incompatible.

If you are always fighting, always arguing, just driving each other crazy, you may have made a mistake by being together.

Some people get married because they believe they are in love, when they were really only in lust. That means that they mistook an initial sexual attraction for long-term compatibility. That, by the way, is an example of how T-chemistry, how surging hormones, can act against your best long-term interest.

We hear these starry-eyed testimonials: "Oh, she's the only person who understands me." Then the same couple goes through an agonizing ten years of marriage, ending in divorce.

They realize years later that they just aren't suited to each other.

It is true in this world that a lot of people were not meant to be together, should probably have just dated, released some body fluids in each other's honor, and then gotten away from each other.

If you find your relationship is beyond repair, if you think that spending years with your partner would be a living death, then get out of the relationship. A long bad relationship will dampen your positive hormonal surges and encourage negative behaviors. You'll end up getting your testosterone rushes in all the wrong ways: anger, irritability, rages, blow-ups, substance dependency, and affairs.

It may be time to let your next relationship be the good one.

These recommendations for couples will help to preserve, protect, and defend a man's precious testosterone chemistry. Couples can then help each other to have happier and more sustained relationships.

17

Spirituality and Health

SPIRITUALITY ENCOURAGES HEALTH and happiness.

A strong spiritual life affects your emotions, which in turn affects your hormones. A faith-rich life can be an added weapon, additional armor, for all the challenges of the modern world.

Rate yourself on this Happiness subsection of the Full T-Questionnaire. Use your score—Mild, Moderate, or Severe—to help determine if there might be a place for spirituality in your life.

——— Your Happiness ———
(10 questions)

1. *Is this you?* "I feel like I was happier and more contented before."

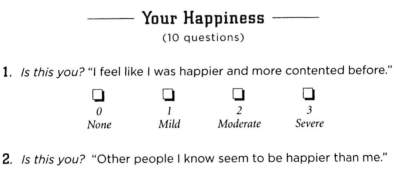

❏	❏	❏	❏
0	*1*	*2*	*3*
None	*Mild*	*Moderate*	*Severe*

2. *Is this you?* "Other people I know seem to be happier than me."

❏	❏	❏	❏
0	*1*	*2*	*3*
None	*Mild*	*Moderate*	*Severe*

3. *Is this you?* "I think that I'll be a burden to others."

❑	❑	❑	❑
0	*1*	*2*	*3*
None	*Mild*	*Moderate*	*Severe*

4. *Is this you?* "There is less laughter and humor in my life."

❑	❑	❑	❑
0	*1*	*2*	*3*
None	*Mild*	*Moderate*	*Severe*

5. *Is this you?* "I seem to be remembering my failures more."

❑	❑	❑	❑
0	*1*	*2*	*3*
None	*Mild*	*Moderate*	*Severe*

6. *Is this you?* "I worry too much."

❑	❑	❑	❑
0	*1*	*2*	*3*
None	*Mild*	*Moderate*	*Severe*

7. *Is this you?* "I'm having bouts of sadness."

❑	❑	❑	❑
0	*1*	*2*	*3*
None	*Mild*	*Moderate*	*Severe*

8. Has the death of a close friend or loved one shaken you, reminding you of your own mortality, that you might be "the next to go"?

❑	❑	❑	❑
0	*1*	*2*	*3*
None	*Mild*	*Moderate*	*Severe*

9. Are you less optimistic about the future?

❑	❑	❑	❑
0	*1*	*2*	*3*
None	*Mild*	*Moderate*	*Severe*

10. *Is this you?* "To everyone else, I have everything going for me, all the outward signs of comfort. But I feel like something's missing, like all these things that I worked so hard to get aren't enough."

❑	❑	❑	❑
0	*1*	*2*	*3*
None	*Mild*	*Moderate*	*Severe*

Your Happiness

Your score:_____/ 30 points

Score/Rating
0 to 3   *None*
4 to 12   *Mild*
13 to 24   *Moderate*
25 to 30   *Severe*

Consider your score range here—is it None, Mild, Moderate, or Severe? Your score will help you determine how you might get some extra benefit from the recommendations in this chapter. While one's happiness and contentment are influenced by many things, men who have a spiritual dimension to their lives do appear to do better.

Assess for yourself if this area can be an added source of strength.

KEEPING THE FAITH

SOME CLIENTS SEE the value of spirituality, and make use of this section. Others dismiss it out of hand. It's a personal decision.

On the one hand, modern medicine doesn't think too highly of faith, belief, or trusting a higher, unseen influence. Doctors cannot detect faith in any of the ways we've been taught. We can't X-ray, MRI, or biopsy faith. We can't cut it in two, surgically remove or implant it, or look at a slice of it under a microscope. We can't weigh it or put it into a bottle, and we don't know the chemical formula. We don't know the optimal dosage, though we have some idea of the side effects. There's no blood test, urine test, DNA analysis, or *faithogram*.

There is, however, compelling research coming out of such institutions as the Center for the Study of Religion, Spirituality and Health at Duke University Medical Center; I would also highly recommend the works of physicians such as Dr. Larry Dossey. Such research affirms the medical value of prayer and the spiritual. It is not so much *what* you believe but *that* you believe that counts. Faith can affect your will, your concentration, and your resilience.

But doctors generally miss out on this powerful capacity of the mind.

Many MDs tell us to stick to hard science, dismissing faith as mythology. So modern medicine dismisses the spiritual side of men. *But . . .*

Key Points

- Faith works. Faith works like a hormone, like medicine.
- Abiding and deep faith builds sources of strength and resilience, including testosterone.

There is compelling evidence that men who lead faith-rich lives do better, whether we're measuring heart attack survival, response to blood pressure medications, wound healing, even cancer survival. Faith-enriched men have an extra buffer against stress and find more meaning and purpose in their lives. Faith even affects your life span: people who never go to a place of worship die about three to five years earlier than those who attend religious services *more* than once per week.

Faith-based programs are gaining more attention. Strengthening people through belief and prayer is being used in:

- Addiction recovery
- Amputation rehabilitation
- Athletic competition
- Burn recovery
- Cancer care
- Chronic pain management
- Combat missions
- Dental pain
- Diabetic sugar control
- Divorce survival
- Emotional abuse recovery
- Grief counseling
- Heart attack survival
- Heart surgery rehabilitation
- HIV care
- Palliative care
- Physical disability
- Recovery from natural disasters such as a hurricane, tsunami, tornado, or earthquake
- Recovery from knee or hip joint replacement surgery
- Serving prison sentences
- Transplant recipients

Why wait till people are dying?

Doctors first discovered the medical value of faith in patients who were terminally ill, who were already on their way out. But why should we only wait till people are dying? How about the living?

In general, men with strong faith-lives respond to medications better, faster, and longer. They need lower doses. They have fewer heart attacks, lower blood pressure, better immune systems, less aggressive cancers, less depression, and they recover from illness quicker.

In fact, I have noted that clients who make use of their spiritual dimension respond faster and more intensely to my testosterone-enrichment program. It seems that men with faith-rich lives have their own chemical source of strength, their own force field, their own firewall.

> MANY TRUE BELIEVERS have complained about the advice I am giving here. They are offended, saying, "You think that religion is just one big exercise in getting your hormones right?"
>
> I can't answer that, but at some level, *everything* can be one big exercise in getting your hormones right.

Researchers are not sure why faith works on the human body. Is it the good Lord above looking after us, or is it part of our own nature that we want to trust in an all-seeing, all-powerful Creator, or both? Is faith just a focused way of using the power of your own mind? Again, it's a personal decision for each man to make.

We call this faith empowerment the "halo effect." Mass delusion or not, it works.

THE HALO EFFECT

Prayer is therapeutic: it's a spiritual form of psychotherapy, self-suggestion, and affirmation.

Deeply felt prayer is known to increase enhancing hormones: melatonin, serotonin, dopamine, beta-endorphins, and testosterone. *Deeply felt prayer* is known to decrease troubling hormones such as cortisol and adrenaline.

> SOME HAVE ASKED, "Is this spirituality effect the same as the placebo effect?" Science cannot perhaps answer that question, but any positive healthful effect is welcome, whatever its source.

WHAT TO DO

- (Re)kindle your faith.
- Pray.
- (Re)join your faith group.
- Have faith in yourself.

(RE)KINDLE YOUR FAITH

"I had lost my way, but I'm trying to get back into it."

Losing your faith? Suddenly feeling you need to believe in something?

That may also be part of a wider midlife change, a midlife reorientation.

Many men who were raised in a home that practiced a faith have since drifted away spiritually. That's fine, probably a healthy sign of growth, skepticism, and questioning. In fact, many of our clients consider themselves too modern to bother with their original beliefs anymore.

But those men who are able to reawaken their spiritual impulses are usually healthier and happier for it.

When they are going through midlife stresses, we encourage men to find all the resources at their disposal and use all the sources of strength they can. Often it is the spouse who drags the reluctant man back into the fold.

If this scenario can work for you, do it.

This Is Not Deep Faith

"DOC, I DID what you said. I had real faith for a whole month, and nothing changed. Nothing seemed to help or make any difference."

In this chapter, I'm talking about deep and abiding faith. The real thing. The whole package.

None of this, "Well, hey, if it works, let me get some of it. . . . Just tell me what you want me to believe, and I'm there."

It's not a bargain. You can't just be a faith-tourist hunting for the benefit.

As one fifty-one-year-old man said, "You see something larger than yourself. You feel like you're part of a tradition . . . a way of dealing with the world. I feel like I'm not alone, like I'm cared for. Like I have access to special mercy, to the ultimate reality."

Men with strong faith:

- Are more optimistic about the future
- Cope better
- Donate to charity more
- Don't abuse substances as much
- Face emergencies more easily
- Feel an added sense of self-respect and worth
- Feel that a higher power is looking out for them
- Feel more secure
- Feel the beauty of nature more
- Feel that eventually they will be going to a better place
- Feel they have some part to play in a master plan
- Feel that there will be some kind of final justice
- Feel that God can work through them
- Find that even suffering can have some kind of purpose or redeeming quality
- Forgive more easily
- Have more powerful, ready, and resilient testosterone

> **FAITH WORKS LIKE a protective umbrella, like a testosterone shield. Basically, belief = medicine.**

PRAY

"I hate my boss. What can I do? I'm more qualified than he is, but he's my boss. Whenever he gets my goat, I go back to my office and read some of our hymns. Or I'll say some of our forgiveness prayers. . . . I think it's the only thing that lets me deal with him."

- Pray for physical health.
- Pray for prosperity.
- Pray for peace of mind.
- Do thankfulness prayers; don't just list demands.

Some places of worship encourage their followers to ask the Higher Force for rather specific things, not just general blessings. It even gets to the point where people will pray for specific mortgage rates, salary increases, grades on tests, the sex of a baby to be born, harm to enemies, and so on.

As a doctor, I believe that more general prayer is more effective, and certainly less disappointing.

Pray for energy, pray for excellence, competence, and the ability to rise to your challenges. Be grateful.

(RE)JOIN YOUR FAITH GROUP

Elvis Presley wore both a cross and a Star of David. He explained, "I didn't want to be shut out of heaven on a technicality."

(Re)joining an organized religion can have many benefits.

Many men have been able to deal with past trauma, abuse, and alcoholism because of the strength they have gotten from fellow members.

They learn elaborate rituals telling them how to get what they want, or at least how to cope with not getting what they want. Much of the benefit also seems to come from having a social network of people with a shared vision.

Men who have strong religious faith usually believe that they are closer to the truth. They believe that their group exclusively is acting on the word of God. This also seems to have an enhancing, T-building effect.

Religious Leaders Are Often Able to help You, as They've Seen It All

Clergy members remind believers that they should forgive, give up grudges, and not seek revenge. The clergy are often asked to help during marriage crises also.

Have Your Congregation Pray for You

Many men feel stronger knowing that their congregation is behind them, praying in their name. So ask fellow members to pray for you. Somehow this works, too.

At some places of worship, they will ask you to specify your problem, arrange for a group prayer, without identifying you by name.

Avoid Negative, Judgmental Congregations

ONE CLIENT WHO was going through T- weakness was told, "You are a sinner. . . . And the reason you have to struggle is that you have sinned against the Lord."

Not exactly a T-boosting source of strength.

Observe Fasting Rituals

Many groups have different types of fasting, staying away from food or drink or sex for particular periods of time. There's a very interesting effect on testosterone. When you start to fast, T goes down, as part of a general conservation effort by the body. But after some time, once you are used to the routine of fasting, there seems to be a general cleansing, a resetting of hormone detectors in the body, and testosterone actually starts rising.

HAVE FAITH IN YOURSELF

"Listen, I'm not particularly religious. . . . I went through some rough patches. First with my parents, who didn't like my wife. Then with my wife, who turned out to be a totally different person than I thought. . . . What keeps me going is the faith I have in myself."

Being spiritual does not necessarily mean being religious, or having to take part in group rituals or services, or consulting regularly with clergymen.

Some clients shy away from organized religion. They are able to add a spiritual dimension to their thinking by believing in themselves, in their own worth, and their own personal purpose. They are not tied to any dogma, religion, or fixed outlook

Speaking with a billionaire in the pharmaceutical industry, I learned of his singular drive. "I started thirty years ago, with two employees and no sales. Now we're global, with five thousand employees, making three billion tablets a month, exporting to seventy countries. For me, it was keeping my eye on the prize, keeping my focus, working toward a goal. I just had faith in myself and my vision."

This type of self-reliant faith also works like a powerful drug.

18

FINAL WORDS

MODERN SOCIETY HAS ADDED YEARS
TO YOUR LIFE—NOW YOU CAN ADD
LIFE TO YOUR YEARS

As you have learned, the master hormone of manhood, testosterone, does a lot. Its first grand performance is at puberty, the coming of age, the onset of manhood. It leads to massive changes in the three areas covered in this book: your physical body, your internal chemistry, and your mind and outlook. Broadening your shoulders, keeping you fertile and ready for sex, keeping you ambitious and valuing companionship—T does all these things.

You've also explored a puzzle that's been troubling doctors and health scientists. If we're all going to live beyond the age of eighty, why don't we live well, in health and with energy? Where does our vitality and vigor go? What's fading once we cross midlife?

As I've hoped to show, part of the answer is fading testosterone. Arguably, there's no single chemical that's as important for a man. This essential hormone basically starts to conk out past the age of forty. And society changes us faster than our biology can keep up. That means we live longer because of many advances—antibiotics, sanitation, vaccines, medical care, and so on. But our bodies and our hormone production capacities have trouble keeping pace.

Then all the negative, unwanted changes start. A bulging stomach, lowered sperm counts and sexual performance, a kind of tired discontent and irritability—a man with diminishing T experiences all these things.

This has real consequences. It's midlife men who start developing epidemics of killer diseases. Heart attacks. High blood pressure. Diabetes. Obesity. Cancer.

Along with actual disease, our quality of life (that famous phrase) also suffers. We have created a modern world that is, it seems, designed to attack all our defenses. Stress. Financial obligations. Poor eating choices. Work politics. Disposable relationships. Nonrestful sleep. Strange, long-term, under-the-radar infections. Most of all, we just don't have *time* for ourselves.

You've also got to think like a doctor. We are familiar with long causes, diseases and problems that develop over years. Let's say you've taken on a mortgage, payments are due monthly, and you're stressed by this. Well, if your stress begins in January, disease and problems don't usually show up by February. It's more of a slow burn, a step-by-step downward spiral, distributed over time. That's why you need to do regular, once-a-year checks, as outlined in this book.

Exactly the same thing, a slow burn, happens with the hormone testosterone. Everything about T suffers. Production is down. Distribution is down. T is challenged. It's ignored. Sent to fight in the wrong location. Overwhelmed by environmental hormones that we eat constantly. It gets soaked up. T even undergoes identity theft—turning into its opposing hormone, estrogen.

Slowly, over years, you basically go through a reverse puberty, a loss of manhood. You lose muscle. Ambition. Energy. And stress tolerance. You become an unwilling prisoner of your own biochemistry. And then you fall into bad habits that temporarily mask these changes but make things worse . . .

Of course, science keeps changing, with new theories and ideas. I look forward to keeping myself, you, and this book up to date with future editions. Then we can all continue to benefit from the latest medical and social research and perspectives.

Nevertheless, what's been so rewarding for me about practicing medicine in this area of men's health for twenty years has been the opportunity to help men. To empower them. To journey together. To bring men to new levels of realization about their own bodies, about what's actually going on under the hood. To share with men practical and (relatively) simple lifestyle choices. To show men and their loved ones that they don't have to fade away after midlife. To show people that heart disease, obesity, irritability, and all the other negatives are not inevitable. And to help men *help doctors* overcome medical blindspots.

In fact, with a little devotion to the program outlined in this book, men can not only *maintain* themselves but also experience an *enhanced* vitality and virility—not just a *rescued* vitality and virility.

To conclude, I say this: Mobilize your own personal testosterone factor. The power is within.

Best wishes,

S. Qaadri, MD

Full
T-Questionnaire

SECTIONS OF THIS T-Questionnaire are distributed throughout this book. Here you will find the entire inventory assembled. It is an elaborate audit and self-assessment of *midlife challenges.*

Warning

If doing the questionnaire all at once:

- Read the guiding comments first.
- Realize that this questionnaire is huge.
- Do it in private.
- Do it honestly.
- Give it adequate time.
- Beware that it highlights strengths, weaknesses, areas of concern, and private matters.

GUIDING COMMENTS

About the Questionnaire

This is a highly detailed, massive inventory of what men may experience after age 40.

It is a lengthy questionnaire. It is *not* a simple magazine-type survey, or a ten-point poll found on the Internet, or from some poster in a doctor's office. Its thorough detail gives it analytical power and medical significance.

There are more questions here than time-pressured MDs will ever get to ask you. Since the average doctor-patient visit lasts less than ten minutes, you will not be able to approach this level of detail when speaking with your health-care practitioner. However, the results of the questionnaire will alert you to what issues may need to be discussed with your physician, so take the time to answer everything and calculate your score.

Doctors recognize patterns; for example, diabetes has a particular pattern of difficulties—excessive thirst, urination, weight loss, and fatigue.

This questionnaire highlights the cluster of symptoms—the pattern—that men may experience in midlife.

It has fifteen sections:

1. Your Changing Body
2. Your Sleep
3. Your Sexuality
4. Your Appearance
5. Your Energy Levels
6. Your Medical Background
7. Your Habits and Lifestyle
8. Your Diet
9. Your Changing Personality
10. Your Mind
11. Your Stress Levels
12. Your Drive
13. Your Self-Esteem
14. Your Relationship
15. Your Happiness

Kinds of Questions

Part of the benefit of this self-inventory is that it gets you thinking about health and well-being issues that we men otherwise may not.

The questions come in various formats. Some concern changes and trends in your physique, habits, personality, feelings, relationships, and sexuality. You are asked what your reactions might be in certain situations, or how much situations apply to your life. Some questions are actual quotations from clients, and you are asked if you agree, and by how much.

The answer grid asks you to rate each question as:

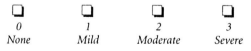

| 0 | 1 | 2 | 3 |
| None | Mild | Moderate | Severe |

Filling out the Questionnaire

Take your time answering the questions.

It's preferable to do the various sections in topical blocks, as they appear in the book. But our advice to clients who want to take the whole questionnaire at once is that they take at least 2½ hours to complete it over two or more sittings. (We don't recommend this, because at a certain stage you may fatigue, not think as clearly as you might, and not give accurate answers.)

Answer honestly—in a way that's truthful, real, for you. Don't give the answers that you think someone else might want or expect to see. Don't withhold answers to personal questions just because someone might be hurt.

Usually, the first response that comes to mind is the real one. Don't overthink and overanalyze, because that can blur your understanding. Don't worry if you think some questions are repetitive, asking the same question from a different angle. Asking similar questions brings out subtle facets of an issue, and also lets that issue count for more. Answer each question with reference to that question only, not on how you may have answered any previous question.

ULTIMATELY, THE QUESTIONNAIRE will provide deeper insight into your health and well-being than most medical appointments or tests.

This questionnaire is the type of inventory we doctors would like to give you, if we had the time, if we had the incentive. But we have neither.

Doctors need to move clients through. We are encouraged to practice high-turnover, efficient, defensive medicine. We are not supposed to devote too much time to any one appointment, or incur costs beyond what's necessary, unless there is a billing motive to the number of tests we order. And that's if you are fortunate enough to have adequate health-care insurance coverage in the first place.

We are watched by insurance companies, reined in by government, wary of trial lawyers, frequently HMO'ed, and "encouraged" by third-party payers in ways that may not always serve our clients' interest.

Generally, we doctors practice *disease* care, not health care. Few payers encourage us to practice preventive medicine. We rescue people from illness and don't generally promote health and well-being.

But this is where you can help yourself—by getting insights into your own health status, with such inventories as the Full T-Questionnaire.

Key Points

- For the man over forty, this detailed questionnaire, honestly answered, usually gives a deeper overall insight into a client's midlife status than most medical appointments or test(s).

- *All* questions are related in some way to testosterone, either directly or indirectly, one or two steps removed.

WHAT TO DO

> THE CHANGES MEASURED here can be spread over ten years or more. That's why you should complete the questionnaire once a year—to measure the progression over time.

- Do the T-Questionnaire sections as they appear in this book. You can also take the entire questionnaire at once here.
- Score each section as you go.
- You may have Severe scores for certain sections. These will alert you to areas of concern.
- For example, many clients discover that the root cause of their midlife difficulties is poor sleep or poor diet.
- Total the overall score.

THE FULL QUESTIONNAIRE

—— Your Changing Body ——
(19 questions)

1. Are you getting overweight, adding a new layer of fat around your waist?

❑	❑	❑	❑
0	*1*	*2*	*3*
None	*Mild*	*Moderate*	*Severe*

2. Are you becoming overweight, developing a double chin?

❑	❑	❑	❑
0	*1*	*2*	*3*
None	*Mild*	*Moderate*	*Severe*

3. Are you catching colds, coughs, and infections more easily?

❑	❑	❑	❑
0	*1*	*2*	*3*
None	*Mild*	*Moderate*	*Severe*

4. Are you developing more allergies—new or worsening asthma, sinus problems, sneezing, or itchy rashes?

❑	❑	❑	❑
0	*1*	*2*	*3*
None	*Mild*	*Moderate*	*Severe*

5. Are you getting more and more skin wrinkles, dry skin, or sagging skin?

❑	❑	❑	❑
0	*1*	*2*	*3*
None	*Mild*	*Moderate*	*Severe*

6. Are flesh wounds healing more slowly?

❑	❑	❑	❑
0	*1*	*2*	*3*
None	*Mild*	*Moderate*	*Severe*

7. Are you rapidly graying or losing your hair?

□	□	□	□
0	*1*	*2*	*3*
None	*Mild*	*Moderate*	*Severe*

8. Is the hair on your legs and chest thinning?

□	□	□	□
0	*1*	*2*	*3*
None	*Mild*	*Moderate*	*Severe*

9. Do you feel you're experiencing more indigestion—more acid, heartburn, bloating, gas?

□	□	□	□
0	*1*	*2*	*3*
None	*Mild*	*Moderate*	*Severe*

10. Are your gums getting swollen and red, bleeding easily when you brush your teeth?

□	□	□	□
0	*1*	*2*	*3*
None	*Mild*	*Moderate*	*Severe*

11. Are your breasts getting bigger, becoming more prominent—almost feminine?

□	□	□	□
0	*1*	*2*	*3*
None	*Mild*	*Moderate*	*Severe*

12. Are your legs and feet getting colder, leading you to wear socks more, even at night?

□	□	□	□
0	*1*	*2*	*3*
None	*Mild*	*Moderate*	*Severe*

13. Are you getting more joint stiffness?

□	□	□	□
0	*1*	*2*	*3*
None	*Mild*	*Moderate*	*Severe*

14. Are your muscles less flexible and more easily strained?

☐	☐	☐	☐
0	*1*	*2*	*3*
None	*Mild*	*Moderate*	*Severe*

15. Are you developing bad posture, slouching, hunching over, and not standing up straight?

☐	☐	☐	☐
0	*1*	*2*	*3*
None	*Mild*	*Moderate*	*Severe*

16. Do you feel like your bones ache deep inside?

☐	☐	☐	☐
0	*1*	*2*	*3*
None	*Mild*	*Moderate*	*Severe*

17. *Is this you?* "I've often got an aching neck, shoulders, or lower back."

☐	☐	☐	☐
0	*1*	*2*	*3*
None	*Mild*	*Moderate*	*Severe*

18. Do you feel your muscle strength is decreasing?

☐	☐	☐	☐
0	*1*	*2*	*3*
None	*Mild*	*Moderate*	*Severe*

19. *Is this you?* "I often ache all over, even though I didn't do that much activity. It's like my body's just been walloped."

☐	☐	☐	☐
0	*1*	*2*	*3*
None	*Mild*	*Moderate*	*Severe*

Your Changing Body

Your score:_____/ 57 points

Score/Rating
0 to 6   *None*
7 to 23   *Mild*
24 to 46 *Moderate*
47 to 57 *Severe*

—— Your Sleep ——
(9 questions)

1. *Is this you?* "I feel like I could always use more sleep."

☐	☐	☐	☐
0	*1*	*2*	*3*
None	*Mild*	*Moderate*	*Severe*

2. *Is this you?* "It doesn't matter how many hours I spend in bed, I'm still not 100 percent the next morning."

☐	☐	☐	☐
0	*1*	*2*	*3*
None	*Mild*	*Moderate*	*Severe*

3. *Does this happen often?* "I put my head on the pillow, and I toss and turn, waiting and waiting to fall asleep."

☐	☐	☐	☐
0	*1*	*2*	*3*
None	*Mild*	*Moderate*	*Severe*

4. *Is this you?* "When I get into bed to sleep, it's hard for me to turn off my thoughts. I've got too much going through my mind."

☐	☐	☐	☐
0	*1*	*2*	*3*
None	*Mild*	*Moderate*	*Severe*

5. *Is this you?* "The slightest little noise or movement wakes me up."

☐	☐	☐	☐
0	*1*	*2*	*3*
None	*Mild*	*Moderate*	*Severe*

6. *Is this you?* "I think I get less than *real* sleep every night."

☐	☐	☐	☐
0	*1*	*2*	*3*
None	*Mild*	*Moderate*	*Severe*

7. Do you wake up often in the middle of the night?

☐	☐	☐	☐
0	*1*	*2*	*3*
None	*Mild*	*Moderate*	*Severe*

8. *Is this you?* "I don't usually remember my dreams."

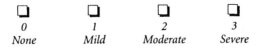

9. *Is this you?* "For me to feel rested, I have to oversleep. I sleep in on the weekends, and get my catch-up rest."

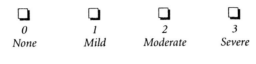

Your Sleep

Your score:_____/ 27 points

Score/Rating

0 to 3   *None*

4 to 11   *Mild*

12 to 22   *Moderate*

23 to 27   *Severe*

——— **Your Sexuality** ———

(21 questions)

Desire

1. Compared to when you were thirty-five, are you having sex less often?

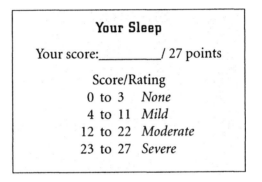

2. *Is this you?* "I'm having sex less often than I would *like*."

3. Are you less horny, have less sexual desire?

4. Do you feel less sexually aroused by your regular partner?

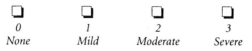

0	1	2	3
None	Mild	Moderate	Severe

Fertility

5. Are you having trouble conceiving either your first or second child because of sperm problems?

0	1	2	3
None	Mild	Moderate	Severe

Erections

6. *Is this you?* "When I used to wake up in the morning, I'd always have an erection. Now, not so much."

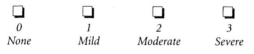

0	1	2	3
None	Mild	Moderate	Severe

7. *Is this you?* "I am *less confident* of getting an erection when I need one, and I worry about my sexual performance."

0	1	2	3
None	Mild	Moderate	Severe

8. Do you feel that your erections are weaker, less full-bodied, less sizable than they were?

0	1	2	3
None	Mild	Moderate	Severe

9. Do you frequently experience difficulty penetrating for sexual intercourse because of weak erections?

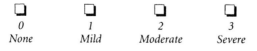

0	1	2	3
None	Mild	Moderate	Severe

10. *Is this you?* "During sex, I often lose my erection."

❑	❑	❑	❑
0	*1*	*2*	*3*
None	*Mild*	*Moderate*	*Severe*

11. Do you ejaculate (come) too soon?

❑	❑	❑	❑
0	*1*	*2*	*3*
None	*Mild*	*Moderate*	*Severe*

12. When you ejaculate, does less fluid come out?

❑	❑	❑	❑
0	*1*	*2*	*3*
None	*Mild*	*Moderate*	*Severe*

13. When you're having an orgasm, do you feel that the muscle contractions, the pulses, are weaker?

❑	❑	❑	❑
0	*1*	*2*	*3*
None	*Mild*	*Moderate*	*Severe*

Satisfaction

14. While you are having sex, are you worried that you might have a heart attack?

❑	❑	❑	❑
0	*1*	*2*	*3*
None	*Mild*	*Moderate*	*Severe*

15. Is your *partner* less sexually satisfied?

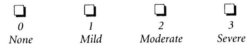

❑	❑	❑	❑
0	*1*	*2*	*3*
None	*Mild*	*Moderate*	*Severe*

16. Have the number or intensity of your *partner's* orgasms lessened?

❑	❑	❑	❑
0	*1*	*2*	*3*
None	*Mild*	*Moderate*	*Severe*

17. Has sex been *less* satisfying for you?

☐
0
None

☐
1
Mild

☐
2
Moderate

☐
3
Severe

18. *Is this you?* "I feel sexually *unsatisfied*."

☐
0
None

☐
1
Mild

☐
2
Moderate

☐
3
Severe

19. Do you find that masturbating, self-pleasuring, is a more intense high than intercourse?

☐
0
None

☐
1
Mild

☐
2
Moderate

☐
3
Severe

20. *Is this you?* "Of course I have orgasms. But they're not as *powerful* anymore. I am not as sensitive down there. It's like I'm thinking, "Yeah, we had sex, but is that it?"

☐
0
None

☐
1
Mild

☐
2
Moderate

☐
3
Severe

21. *Is this you?* "Sexually, I was always ready to go, ready to rock. But now we've got to do all this stuff to get me up and going—I need a lot more stimulation. I really miss the old days. Where's the magic gone?"

☐
0
None

☐
1
Mild

☐
2
Moderate

☐
3
Severe

Your Sexuality

Your score:_____/ 63 points

Score/Rating

0 to 6   *None*

7 to 25   *Mild*

26 to 50 *Moderate*

51 to 63 *Severe*

——— Your Appearance ———
(5 questions)

1. Are you less pleased about how you look?

☐	☐	☐	☐
0	*1*	*2*	*3*
None	*Mild*	*Moderate*	*Severe*

2. Are you less concerned with grooming, with your facial hair and hairstyle?

☐	☐	☐	☐
0	*1*	*2*	*3*
None	*Mild*	*Moderate*	*Severe*

3. *Is this you?* "I used to get more positive attention because of my physical appearance, and this bothers me."

☐	☐	☐	☐
0	*1*	*2*	*3*
None	*Mild*	*Moderate*	*Severe*

4. Have you seriously thought about plastic surgery to enhance your self-image?

☐	☐	☐	☐
0	*1*	*2*	*3*
None	*Mild*	*Moderate*	*Severe*

5. Are you concerned that you're looking *too old too fast*, aging before your time?

☐	☐	☐	☐
0	*1*	*2*	*3*
None	*Mild*	*Moderate*	*Severe*

Your Appearance

Your score:_____/ 15 points

Score/Rating
0 to 2   *None*
3 to 6   *Mild*
7 to 12 *Moderate*
13 to 15 *Severe*

——— Your Energy Levels ———
(5 questions)

1. Are you feeling lazier, with less get-up-and-go?

❑	❑	❑	❑
0	*1*	*2*	*3*
None	*Mild*	*Moderate*	*Severe*

2. Do you fatigue quickly?

❑	❑	❑	❑
0	*1*	*2*	*3*
None	*Mild*	*Moderate*	*Severe*

3. *Is this you?* "I fall asleep when I don't mean to—when I'm watching TV, or right after dinner."

❑	❑	❑	❑
0	*1*	*2*	*3*
None	*Mild*	*Moderate*	*Severe*

4. Do you *feel* older than your actual age?

❑	❑	❑	❑
0	*1*	*2*	*3*
None	*Mild*	*Moderate*	*Severe*

5. *Is this you?* "My stamina has really gone down over the last couple of years."

❑	❑	❑	❑
0	*1*	*2*	*3*
None	*Mild*	*Moderate*	*Severe*

Your Energy Levels

Your score:＿＿＿＿＿/ 15 points

Score/Rating

0 to 2	*None*
3 to 6	*Mild*
7 to 12	*Moderate*
13 to 15	*Severe*

——— Your Medical Background ———
(14 questions)

1. *Is this you?* "I smoke cigarettes daily."

    ☐   ☐   ☐   ☐
    0   *1*   *2*   *3*
    None   *Mild*   *Moderate*   *Severe*

2. Have you been particularly exposed to chemicals—such as solvents, industrial fumes, cleaners, pesticides, herbicides, or petroleum products?

    ☐   ☐   ☐   ☐
    0   *1*   *2*   *3*
    None   *Mild*   *Moderate*   *Severe*

3. *Is this you?* "I have had groin hernia(s) and or mumps."

    ☐   ☐   ☐   ☐
    0   *1*   *2*   *3*
    None   *Mild*   *Moderate*   *Severe*

4. Do you have a close male relative who died of cancer?

    ☐   ☐   ☐   ☐
    0   *1*   *2*   *3*
    None   *Mild*   *Moderate*   *Severe*

5. During your childhood, were you verbally, physically, or sexually abused?

    ☐   ☐   ☐   ☐
    0   *1*   *2*   *3*
    None   *Mild*   *Moderate*   *Severe*

6. *Is this you?* "I have been diagnosed with depression at some time in my life."

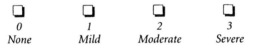

    ☐   ☐   ☐   ☐
    0   *1*   *2*   *3*
    None   *Mild*   *Moderate*   *Severe*

7. *Is this you?* "I am obese, really overweight."

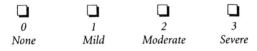

    ☐   ☐   ☐   ☐
    0   *1*   *2*   *3*
    None   *Mild*   *Moderate*   *Severe*

8. Do you have a close male relative who had a heart attack?

☐	☐	☐	☐
0	*1*	*2*	*3*
None	*Mild*	*Moderate*	*Severe*

9. *Is this you?* "I have heart disease."

☐	☐	☐	☐
0	*1*	*2*	*3*
None	*Mild*	*Moderate*	*Severe*

10. *Is this you?* "A number of male members of my family have died before age 50."

☐	☐	☐	☐
0	*1*	*2*	*3*
None	*Mild*	*Moderate*	*Severe*

11. *Is this you?* "I have high blood pressure."

☐	☐	☐	☐
0	*1*	*2*	*3*
None	*Mild*	*Moderate*	*Severe*

12. *Is this you?* "I have high cholesterol."

☐	☐	☐	☐
0	*1*	*2*	*3*
None	*Mild*	*Moderate*	*Severe*

13. *Is this you?* "I have diabetes."

☐	☐	☐	☐
0	*1*	*2*	*3*
None	*Mild*	*Moderate*	*Severe*

14. *Is this you?* "Even if I scored very high on this questionnaire, I don't have a health-care practitioner who I feel would really help me.

"My doctor won't take the time to discuss all of my needs, and I don't feel all that comfortable opening up to him, anyway. He might just brush me off by prescribing a sleeping pill or Viagra, or some other drug. He might just tell me to get used to the idea of getting old."

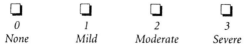

☐	☐	☐	☐
0	*1*	*2*	*3*
None	*Mild*	*Moderate*	*Severe*

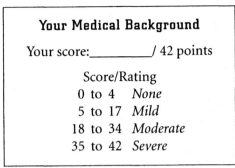

———— Your Habits and Lifestyle ————

(11 questions)

1. *Is this you?* "I have spent my whole life meeting deadlines."

❑	❑	❑	❑
0	*1*	*2*	*3*
None	*Mild*	*Moderate*	*Severe*

2. Do you have too many late nights?

❑	❑	❑	❑
0	*1*	*2*	*3*
None	*Mild*	*Moderate*	*Severe*

3. *Is this you?* "I do little, if any, exercise."

❑	❑	❑	❑
0	*1*	*2*	*3*
None	*Mild*	*Moderate*	*Severe*

4. *Is this you?* "Over the years, it seems I've devoted too much time and emotion to my work, and not enough to my home life."

❑	❑	❑	❑
0	*1*	*2*	*3*
None	*Mild*	*Moderate*	*Severe*

5. Do you think, "Who has the time to exercise?"

❑	❑	❑	❑
0	*1*	*2*	*3*
None	*Mild*	*Moderate*	*Severe*

6. Do you think, "Who has the time for all those positive, healthy lifestyle changes they keep talking about?"

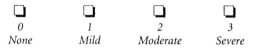

| 0 | 1 | 2 | 3 |
| *None* | *Mild* | *Moderate* | *Severe* |

7. Did you have a lot of sexual partners in your life?

| 0 | 1 | 2 | 3 |
| *None* | *Mild* | *Moderate* | *Severe* |

8. *Is this you?* If your wife or partner suggests you get a health check-up, you reply, "Look, I'm fine. There's nothing wrong with me. It'll go away on its own. Let's just forget about it."

| 0 | 1 | 2 | 3 |
| *None* | *Mild* | *Moderate* | *Severe* |

9. *Is this you?* "I don't have access to good health care."

| 0 | 1 | 2 | 3 |
| *None* | *Mild* | *Moderate* | *Severe* |

10. *Is this you?* "Yes, sure, I watch a lot of TV. And I spend a lot of time on the computer too, on the Internet. I find it relaxing."

| 0 | 1 | 2 | 3 |
| *None* | *Mild* | *Moderate* | *Severe* |

11. *Is this you?* "I don't belong to any particular faith. I don't believe in all that religious stuff. There's no higher power, so what's the point of praying? It's just us."

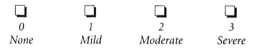

| 0 | 1 | 2 | 3 |
| *None* | *Mild* | *Moderate* | *Severe* |

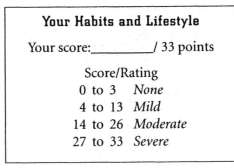

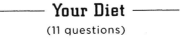

—— Your Diet ——
(11 questions)

1. *Is this you?* "I've heard of but don't follow all those 'health' diets."

❑	❑	❑	❑
0	*1*	*2*	*3*
None	*Mild*	*Moderate*	*Severe*

2. *Is this you?* "I pretty well eat whatever I want, whenever I like."

❑	❑	❑	❑
0	*1*	*2*	*3*
None	*Mild*	*Moderate*	*Severe*

3. *Is this you?* "I like to snack daily on chips, candies, cookies, or popcorn—just about any munchies."

❑	❑	❑	❑
0	*1*	*2*	*3*
None	*Mild*	*Moderate*	*Severe*

4. *Is this you?* "I have more than two alcoholic drinks of per day."

❑	❑	❑	❑
0	*1*	*2*	*3*
None	*Mild*	*Moderate*	*Severe*

5. *Is this you?* "I have more than two caffeinated drinks per day."

❑	❑	❑	❑
0	*1*	*2*	*3*
None	*Mild*	*Moderate*	*Severe*

6. *Is this you?* "I eat a lot of salt."

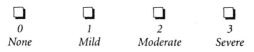

	0	1	2	3
	None	Mild	Moderate	Severe

7. Is your evening timetable for food and relaxation dictated by the TV program schedule?

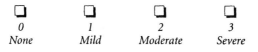

	0	1	2	3
	None	Mild	Moderate	Severe

8. *Is this you?* "I don't like the idea of taking pills, and I can't bring myself to take vitamins or supplements regularly."

	0	1	2	3
	None	Mild	Moderate	Severe

9. Do you regularly skip meals, perhaps having only one or two meals per day?

	0	1	2	3
	None	Mild	Moderate	Severe

10. Do you wonder, "Why does food that's healthy taste so bad, so *blah*? Even a rabbit would get tired of it."

	0	1	2	3
	None	Mild	Moderate	Severe

11. *Is this you?* "Take care of my nutrition? With the amount of money I spend on junk food, I am personally supporting the fast-food industry. I'm a junk-food junkie."

Your Diet

Your score:_____/ 33 points

Score/Rating

0 to 3   *None*

4 to 13 *Mild*

14 to 26 *Moderate*

27 to 33 *Severe*

—— Your Changing Personality ——
(11 questions)

1. Do you blame others more?

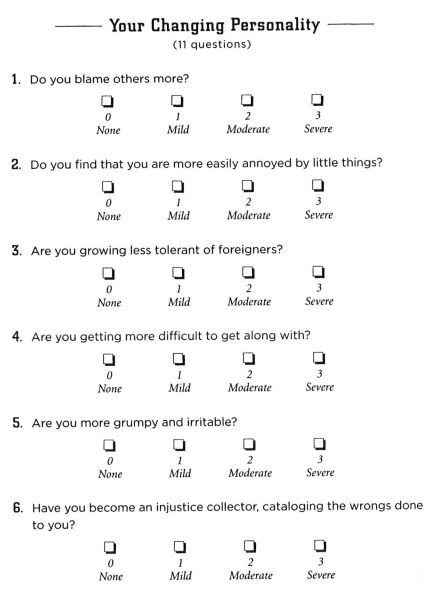

❑	❑	❑	❑
0	*1*	*2*	*3*
None	*Mild*	*Moderate*	*Severe*

2. Do you find that you are more easily annoyed by little things?

❑	❑	❑	❑
0	*1*	*2*	*3*
None	*Mild*	*Moderate*	*Severe*

3. Are you growing less tolerant of foreigners?

❑	❑	❑	❑
0	*1*	*2*	*3*
None	*Mild*	*Moderate*	*Severe*

4. Are you getting more difficult to get along with?

❑	❑	❑	❑
0	*1*	*2*	*3*
None	*Mild*	*Moderate*	*Severe*

5. Are you more grumpy and irritable?

❑	❑	❑	❑
0	*1*	*2*	*3*
None	*Mild*	*Moderate*	*Severe*

6. Have you become an injustice collector, cataloging the wrongs done to you?

❑	❑	❑	❑
0	*1*	*2*	*3*
None	*Mild*	*Moderate*	*Severe*

7. Do you have a shorter fuse, and blow up more frequently?

❑	❑	❑	❑
0	*1*	*2*	*3*
None	*Mild*	*Moderate*	*Severe*

8. Do your loved ones wonder why you're more resentful and hostile?

❑	❑	❑	❑
0	*1*	*2*	*3*
None	*Mild*	*Moderate*	*Severe*

9. *Is this you?* "I find myself feeling insulted more easily."

❑	❑	❑	❑
0	*1*	*2*	*3*
None	*Mild*	*Moderate*	*Severe*

10. Do you find yourself wishing revenge on your enemies more often?

❑	❑	❑	❑
0	*1*	*2*	*3*
None	*Mild*	*Moderate*	*Severe*

11. *Is this you?* On the road, another driver cuts in front of you. Your temper flares, you rage, shout insults, give him the finger, and wish you could nuke the guy off the face of the earth.

❑	❑	❑	❑
0	*1*	*2*	*3*
None	*Mild*	*Moderate*	*Severe*

Your Changing Personality:

Your score:_____/ 33 points

Score/Rating
0 to 3   *None*
4 to 13 *Mild*
14 to 26 *Moderate*
27 to 33 *Severe*

——— Your Mind ———
(6 questions)

1. Is your thinking not as sharp, not as clear?

❑	❑	❑	❑
0	*1*	*2*	*3*
None	*Mild*	*Moderate*	*Severe*

2. Do you feel less creative, stuck for new ideas?

❑	❑	❑	❑
0	*1*	*2*	*3*
None	*Mild*	*Moderate*	*Severe*

3. *Is this you?* "I notice some difficulty from time to time searching for the right word."

❑	❑	❑	❑
0	*1*	*2*	*3*
None	*Mild*	*Moderate*	*Severe*

4. *Is this you?* "I find that learning new information is more of a struggle."

❑	❑	❑	❑
0	*1*	*2*	*3*
None	*Mild*	*Moderate*	*Severe*

5. *Is this you?* "I find that I'm less able to figure things out, less able to analyze problems. I'm slower on the uptake."

❑	❑	❑	❑
0	*1*	*2*	*3*
None	*Mild*	*Moderate*	*Severe*

6. *Is this you?* "I considered myself a pretty good thinker. But I'm not as decisive as I was before, and my attention span is shorter. I wonder if my memory is weakening."

❑	❑	❑	❑
0	*1*	*2*	*3*
None	*Mild*	*Moderate*	*Severe*

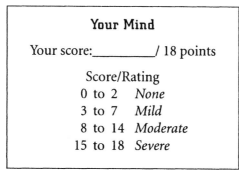

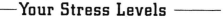

Your Stress Levels

(9 questions)

1. *Is this you?* "I'm feeling the load of too many responsibilities, and they keep coming."

❑	❑	❑	❑
0	*1*	*2*	*3*
None	*Mild*	*Moderate*	*Severe*

2. Does your personality clash with that of your boss or supervisor?

❑	❑	❑	❑
0	*1*	*2*	*3*
None	*Mild*	*Moderate*	*Severe*

3. *Is this you?* "My home environment stresses me out frequently."

❑	❑	❑	❑
0	*1*	*2*	*3*
None	*Mild*	*Moderate*	*Severe*

4. *Is this you?* "The politics at work are such a headache."

❑	❑	❑	❑
0	*1*	*2*	*3*
None	*Mild*	*Moderate*	*Severe*

5. Do you often think, "Please, let me win the lottery so I can get the heck away from all that I have to deal with"?

❑	❑	❑	❑
0	*1*	*2*	*3*
None	*Mild*	*Moderate*	*Severe*

6. *Is this you?* "I would truly benefit from more regular vacation time."

☐	☐	☐	☐
0	*1*	*2*	*3*
None	*Mild*	*Moderate*	*Severe*

7. Do you feel like you're not performing at your best, and having more "off days"?

☐	☐	☐	☐
0	*1*	*2*	*3*
None	*Mild*	*Moderate*	*Severe*

8. *Is this you?* "To release stress, to relax, I'm turning to unhealthy practices—like drinking, smoking, or overeating. I know it's not good for me, but that's how I take the edge off."

☐	☐	☐	☐
0	*1*	*2*	*3*
None	*Mild*	*Moderate*	*Severe*

9. *Is this you?* "I often feel like I'm rushing from one activity to the next. I wonder if I'd qualify for this new condition they're talking about, 'hurried-man syndrome'?"

☐	☐	☐	☐
0	*1*	*2*	*3*
None	*Mild*	*Moderate*	*Severe*

Your Stress Levels:

Your score:_____/ 27 points

Score/Rating
0 to 3 *None*
4 to 11 *Mild*
12 to 22 *Moderate*
23 to 27 *Severe*

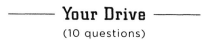

Your Drive
(10 questions)

1. Are you less enthusiastic about *home* activities and projects that used to stir your imagination?

☐	☐	☐	☐
0	*1*	*2*	*3*
None	*Mild*	*Moderate*	*Severe*

2. Are you less eager about *work* activities and projects that used to stir your imagination?

☐	☐	☐	☐
0	*1*	*2*	*3*
None	*Mild*	*Moderate*	*Severe*

3. When completing a task or project, do you settle for what's adequate, not for the best that you can do?

☐	☐	☐	☐
0	*1*	*2*	*3*
None	*Mild*	*Moderate*	*Severe*

4. *Is this you?* "I'm not so motivated to take on new challenges. I'm comfortable in my settled ways."

☐	☐	☐	☐
0	*1*	*2*	*3*
None	*Mild*	*Moderate*	*Severe*

5. *Is this you?* "I don't feel so ambitious at work anymore. I feel blocked."

☐	☐	☐	☐
0	*1*	*2*	*3*
None	*Mild*	*Moderate*	*Severe*

6. *Is this you?* "I'm not as self-confident as before."

☐	☐	☐	☐
0	*1*	*2*	*3*
None	*Mild*	*Moderate*	*Severe*

7. *Is this you?* "I pursue fewer social engagements and make fewer good friends now."

❑	❑	❑	❑
0	*1*	*2*	*3*
None	*Mild*	*Moderate*	*Severe*

8. *Is this you?* "Before, I felt like I had four-wheel drive. Now, I'm not so sure."

❑	❑	❑	❑
0	*1*	*2*	*3*
None	*Mild*	*Moderate*	*Severe*

9. *Is this you?* "I do live with the possibility of losing my job, of being downsized. It can be quite disheartening."

❑	❑	❑	❑
0	*1*	*2*	*3*
None	*Mild*	*Moderate*	*Severe*

10. At work, do you think, "God, how many more years do I have to do this?"

❑	❑	❑	❑
0	*1*	*2*	*3*
None	*Mild*	*Moderate*	*Severe*

11. *Is this you?* "I feel somewhat intimidated by the younger guys at work. It's like they're ready to take over, to displace me. That saps your dedication."

❑	❑	❑	❑
0	*1*	*2*	*3*
None	*Mild*	*Moderate*	*Severe*

Your Drive

Your score:_____ / 30 points

Score/Rating

0 to 3	*None*
4 to 12	*Mild*
13 to 24	*Moderate*
25 to 30	*Severe*

──── Your Self-Esteem ────
(10 questions)

1. Do you feel what you contribute to your *household* is taken for granted, and not appreciated enough?

❑	❑	❑	❑
0	*1*	*2*	*3*
None	*Mild*	*Moderate*	*Severe*

2. Do you feel what you contribute to your *workplace* is taken for granted, and not appreciated enough?

❑	❑	❑	❑
0	*1*	*2*	*3*
None	*Mild*	*Moderate*	*Severe*

3. "I think there's less opportunity for me to advance now. This is making me bitter."

❑	❑	❑	❑
0	*1*	*2*	*3*
None	*Mild*	*Moderate*	*Severe*

4. Do you feel you are making less money than you're worth?

❑	❑	❑	❑
0	*1*	*2*	*3*
None	*Mild*	*Moderate*	*Severe*

5. *Is this you?* "I think that I have passed my peak."

❑	❑	❑	❑
0	*1*	*2*	*3*
None	*Mild*	*Moderate*	*Severe*

6. *Is this you?* "I thought I would own more by now."

❑	❑	❑	❑
0	*1*	*2*	*3*
None	*Mild*	*Moderate*	*Severe*

7. Is it important to you that your favorite sports team(s) win?

❑	❑	❑	❑
0	*1*	*2*	*3*
None	*Mild*	*Moderate*	*Severe*

8. Do your kids or colleagues joke that you are definitely part of the older generation?

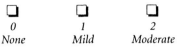

| 0 | 1 | 2 | 3 |
| *None* | *Mild* | *Moderate* | *Severe* |

9. *Is this you?* "I feel that my contemporaries and colleagues get ahead and get promoted faster than me. I feel cheated."

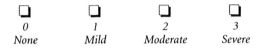

| 0 | 1 | 2 | 3 |
| *None* | *Mild* | *Moderate* | *Severe* |

10. *Is this you?* "You try and do right by your kids. You give them everything they need . . . love, everything. But what happens? I have to say, my kids disappoint me. They haven't lived up to my expectations."

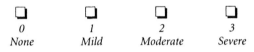

| 0 | 1 | 2 | 3 |
| *None* | *Mild* | *Moderate* | *Severe* |

Your Self-Esteem

Your score:_____/ 30 points

Score/Rating
0 to 3   *None*
4 to 12   *Mild*
13 to 24   *Moderate*
25 to 30   *Severe*

———— Your Relationship ————
(16 questions)

1. Are you losing the affection and romance in your relationship?

☐	☐	☐	☐
0	*1*	*2*	*3*
None	*Mild*	*Moderate*	*Severe*

2. *Is this you?* "I'm getting less out of my relationship than I put into it."

☐	☐	☐	☐
0	*1*	*2*	*3*
None	*Mild*	*Moderate*	*Severe*

3. Do you feel you're in a bad relationship?

☐	☐	☐	☐
0	*1*	*2*	*3*
None	*Mild*	*Moderate*	*Severe*

4. Do you regularly think about getting out of your relationship?

☐	☐	☐	☐
0	*1*	*2*	*3*
None	*Mild*	*Moderate*	*Severe*

5. Do you forgive less?

☐	☐	☐	☐
0	*1*	*2*	*3*
None	*Mild*	*Moderate*	*Severe*

6. *Is this you?* "When we disagree, it often turns into an argument. We don't seem to be able to disagree in a mature, civilized manner."

☐	☐	☐	☐
0	*1*	*2*	*3*
None	*Mild*	*Moderate*	*Severe*

7. *Is this you?* "We argue too frequently."

☐	☐	☐	☐
0	*1*	*2*	*3*
None	*Mild*	*Moderate*	*Severe*

8. When you argue, do you explode like a volcano, hurling insults at your partner?

❑	❑	❑	❑
0	*1*	*2*	*3*
None	*Mild*	*Moderate*	*Severe*

9. *Is this you?* "When my kids were young, they slept in our bed, right up until they were about five or six years old."

❑	❑	❑	❑
0	*1*	*2*	*3*
None	*Mild*	*Moderate*	*Severe*

10. If you have a fight, can a lot of time go by without speaking to each other—because of a domestic cold war?

❑	❑	❑	❑
0	*1*	*2*	*3*
None	*Mild*	*Moderate*	*Severe*

11. Do you think about having an affair, and wish you had the guts to have one?

❑	❑	❑	❑
0	*1*	*2*	*3*
None	*Mild*	*Moderate*	*Severe*

12. *Is this you?* "I am ready to *receive* affection, but I don't give it so much."

❑	❑	❑	❑
0	*1*	*2*	*3*
None	*Mild*	*Moderate*	*Severe*

13. Does your partner feel you're married to your computer?

❑	❑	❑	❑
0	*1*	*2*	*3*
None	*Mild*	*Moderate*	*Severe*

14. *Is this you?* "I don't know why, but I remember my old girlfriends more, even the ones who got away. They'll just pop into my mind—memories of some of my encounters from earlier days."

❑	❑	❑	❑
0	*1*	*2*	*3*
None	*Mild*	*Moderate*	*Severe*

15. *Is this you?* "I don't get the support I need from my partner. I'll suggest some idea or scheme, and I'll get one of those *here-we-go-again* looks."

❏	❏	❏	❏
0	*1*	*2*	*3*
None	*Mild*	*Moderate*	*Severe*

16. *Is this you?* Your partner wants *to talk,* and asks how your day was. You're thinking, "Oh God, give it a rest, will you? Just leave me alone." You give brush-off replies, "Fine, yeah, everything's fine. Nothing's wrong."

❏	❏	❏	❏
0	*1*	*2*	*3*
None	*Mild*	*Moderate*	*Severe*

Your Relationship

Your score:_____/ 48 points

Score/Rating
0 to 5   *None*
6 to 19   *Mild*
20 to 38   *Moderate*
39 to 48   *Severe*

——— Your Happiness ———
(10 questions)

1. *Is this you?* "I feel like I was happier and more contented before."

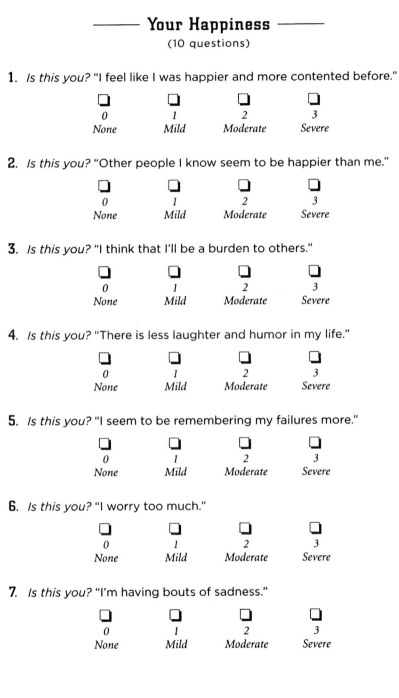

❑	❑	❑	❑
0	*1*	*2*	*3*
None	*Mild*	*Moderate*	*Severe*

2. *Is this you?* "Other people I know seem to be happier than me."

❑	❑	❑	❑
0	*1*	*2*	*3*
None	*Mild*	*Moderate*	*Severe*

3. *Is this you?* "I think that I'll be a burden to others."

❑	❑	❑	❑
0	*1*	*2*	*3*
None	*Mild*	*Moderate*	*Severe*

4. *Is this you?* "There is less laughter and humor in my life."

❑	❑	❑	❑
0	*1*	*2*	*3*
None	*Mild*	*Moderate*	*Severe*

5. *Is this you?* "I seem to be remembering my failures more."

❑	❑	❑	❑
0	*1*	*2*	*3*
None	*Mild*	*Moderate*	*Severe*

6. *Is this you?* "I worry too much."

❑	❑	❑	❑
0	*1*	*2*	*3*
None	*Mild*	*Moderate*	*Severe*

7. *Is this you?* "I'm having bouts of sadness."

❑	❑	❑	❑
0	*1*	*2*	*3*
None	*Mild*	*Moderate*	*Severe*

8. Has the death of a close friend or loved one shaken you, reminding you of your own mortality, that you might be the next to go?

❑	❑	❑	❑
0	*1*	*2*	*3*
None	*Mild*	*Moderate*	*Severe*

9. Are you less optimistic about the future?

❑	❑	❑	❑
0	*1*	*2*	*3*
None	*Mild*	*Moderate*	*Severe*

10. *Is this you?* "To everyone else, I have everything going for me, all the outward signs of comfort. But I feel like something's missing, like all these things that I worked so hard to get aren't enough."

❑	❑	❑	❑
0	*1*	*2*	*3*
None	*Mild*	*Moderate*	*Severe*

Your Happiness

Your score:_____/ 30 points

Score/Rating
0 to 3   *None*
4 to 12   *Mild*
13 to 24   *Moderate*
25 to 30   *Severe*

Full T-Questionnaire Scoring Sheet

WRITE **YOUR SCORES** from each section of the T-Questionnaire here. The maximum scores for each section are also shown.

SECTION	INDIVIDUAL SECTION SCORES
Your Changing Body	_____ / 57 Points
Your Sleep	_____ / 27 Points
Your Sexuality	_____ / 63 Points
Your Appearance	_____ / 15 Points
Your Energy Levels	_____ / 15 Points
Your Medical Background	_____ / 42 Points
Your Habits and Lifestyle	_____ / 33 Points
Your Diet	_____ / 33 Points
Your Changing Personality	_____ / 33 Points
Your Mind	_____ / 18 Points
Your Stress Levels	_____ / 27 Points
Your Drive	_____ / 30 Points
Your Self-Esteem	_____ / 30 Points
Your Relationship	_____ / 48 Points
Your Happiness	_____ / 30 Points
Grand total of all sections =	_____ / 500 Points

Appendix C discusses the meaning of the grand total in detail.

Full T-Questionnaire Scoring Explanation

THIS CHAPTER IS an explanation of your *overall score*.

Key Points

- The Full T-Questionnaire ties together the many isolated, separate, and less easily measured signs and events in the lives of midlife men.
- Your score range—Mild, Moderate, or Severe—alerts you to the intensity of the midlife challenges you are experiencing.
- Your score is a guide to how intensely you should follow the core material in this book, helping you to enhance and extend your vitality and virility.

WHAT TO DO

- Add up your overall Full T-Questionnaire score.
- Understand the general numbers.
- Graph your score.
- Understand the categories.
- Understand the nuances about this questionnaire and its scoring.
- Follow all the chapters, but pay special attention to the core recommendations based on your score.
- Take the Full T-Questionnaire once a year to monitor changes and your drifting score.

ADD UP YOUR OVERALL FULL T-QUESTIONNAIRE SCORE

The maximum score is 500 points.

Scoring	
0 to 50	*None*
50 to 200	*Mild*
200 to 400	*Moderate*
400 to 500	*Severe*

For example, if your total was 190 points, you would be in the Mild range, 50 to 200 points.

But what does this score measure? Mild, Moderate, or Severe *what?*

This is a questionnaire about *midlife challenges.* More formally, it is a questionnaire about andropause, a kind of menopause that men experience. *Androgens* is the broad name for the many testosterone-like substances produced in a man's body, thus the term *andropause.*

Helping baby-boomer men is a relatively new field, so the labels are still being hotly debated. Midlife challenges have been called many things, from "the midlife crisis" and andropause to hypotestosteronemia (low-blood testosterone) and partial androgen deficiency in the aging male (PADAM). Whatever term you prefer, these labels stand for the chemical and personality changes that act as a drag on a man's physique, behavior, emotions, thinking, energy, drive, ambition, and sexuality.

These are the changes that rob men over forty of their vitality and virility.

Terminology Overload

ULTIMATELY, THIS BOOK is about helping men anticipate, cope with, alleviate and reverse midlife changes. It is about helping men extend their prime of life. It's also about enhancing well-being and health. We are not so concerned about terminology, so don't get hung up on the words.

Doctors spend a lot of time devising high-sounding words, some of which add value, some of which look plausible on billing forms.

A good elaboration of the symptoms of andropause—the midlife challenges, what men over forty go through—is the questionnaire itself.

UNDERSTAND THE GENERAL NUMBERS

Men over forty who take this questionnaire, in our experience, fall into the following scoring divisions:

SCORE	CATEGORY	PERCENTAGE OF MEN
0 to 50	None	10%
50 to 200	Mild	45%
200 to 400	Moderate	35%
400 to 500	Severe	10%

The pie-chart graph looks like this:

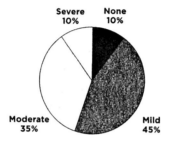

How men over forty score on the questionnaire.

This is the distribution for the clients that I see. No doubt, the numbers would be somewhat different if this questionnaire were given to *all* men over forty.

Where Do You Stand?

Are you like most men, in the Mild category? Among the fortunate 10 percent who have few concerns, the None category? Or in the higher-end categories, Moderate or Severe?

Some male clients give me two questionnaires: the one that their partner "helped" them complete, and the real one. They tell me that they couldn't, for example, answer the Sexuality or Relationship questionnaire sections honestly, because of scrutiny at home.

Your Real Answers, Please

MEN ARE AN interesting lot. Even when a doctor offers them a health questionnaire, to be completed in private, some men fudge the answers. They give doctors answers that they think we want, or that they think we should hear. Answer in a way that's appropriate, real, and honest for you.

My advice is not to misrepresent yourself to either your lawyer, because he or she will do that for you, or to your health-care practitioner, because it is nonproductive.

GRAPH YOUR SCORE

"Doc, it's revealing to see how my score can change over time."

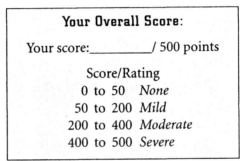

Your Overall Score:

Your score:_____/ 500 points

Score/Rating
0 to 50   *None*
50 to 200   *Mild*
200 to 400   *Moderate*
400 to 500   *Severe*

Visualize the information.

We ask our clients to graph their results from year to year on the same paper. This graphic version helps them to visually monitor changes, improvements, and declines. This drawn record then becomes a snapshot of their life experience over time.

On the following bar graph, draw a line where your score would be, labeling it with the month and year that you took the test, such as *June 2006*:

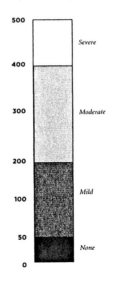

For example,

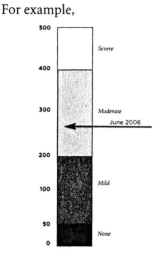

If you took the test in June 2006, scoring 300 points, you would draw a straight line through the bar graph as shown.

UNDERSTAND THE CATEGORIES

Here is a more detailed description of each scoring division.

☑	☐	☐	☐
0	*1*	*2*	*3*
None	*Mild*	*Moderate*	*Severe*

Score: 0 to 50 None

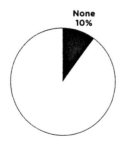

Fantastic. This is remarkable. Ten percent of our clients are here.

If your score is between 0 and 50, keep up the good work, attitude, and habits. You're there. You are already functioning at your prime of life, with full vitality and virility. You may have a few issues, but nothing too worrisome.

It means in all the major areas that concern men over forty, you're doing extremely well: physique, sleep, energy, self-esteem, stress levels, sexuality, energy, drive, and so on.

Nevertheless, this book can still help you by alerting you to oncoming life changes. By knowing how to recognize, prevent, and manage problems early, you will be doing your body and mind a great service.

Another group of men who score in this category are those who have worked their way into it. Initially, these men would have scored in the higher, troubled categories—Mild, Moderate, or Severe. Then they followed the regimen in this book. They improved themselves and their scores dropped.

Regardless of how you made your way into this excellent, highly functioning category, congratulations.

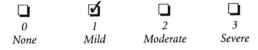

Score: 50 to 200 Mild

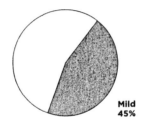

This is the most common category.

Good. About 45 percent of the midlife men I see score in the Mild range.

This is a broad category, but a hopeful one. It means, "Okay, things are still good, there are a number of concerns, but you've recognized this early. You didn't allow things to slide too much."

A man in the Mild category is still fine, functioning, and participating in life. He's still walking around, but he's not at his very best, not at his prime, not at his maximum vitality and virility. He likely will not realize that he's troubled by so many complaints, unless he goes through a vigorous self-assessment such as the Full T-Questionnaire.

And like most men, he'll just drift through life without making any proactive, positive lifestyle changes. He'll let his score coast upward—deteriorate—by about 25 to 100 points every year. Eventually, he'll be out of the Mild range.

Slowly, over years, he will accumulate more and more of the midlife difficulties detailed in the questionnaire.

A Salute to Baby-Boomer Men

THERE IS ANOTHER valuable and vocal subgroup of men who score in the Mild to Moderate ranges. In our experience, these men are executives, elected members of government, managers, commercial artists, and knowledge workers.

These men demand more out of life. They are very concerned about optimizing their health, work performance, business success, and creative output, but they feel that there's a drag on their efforts. Whatever they try doesn't work to their satisfaction.

They then vigorously apply the lessons in this book, and self-optimize.

This is a group of baby-boomer men who are leading social change. By their own example, they are teaching other men how to revitalize themselves, and they are forcing health-care practitioners and the medical establishment to respond to their needs with more than just pills.

There is a wide range of scores in the Mild category:

50 to 100 low-Mild
100 to 150 mid-Mild
150 to 200 high-Mild

If you scored just above 50, you are very near your prime, your optimal level of functioning. This is a *low*-Mild score. You should be able to improve (drop your score) with relatively modest effort.

On the other hand, if you scored just below 200—say, 190—you are almost in the Moderate range. This is a high-Mild score. You must realize that with time, without any lifestyle changes, you will almost certainly deteriorate or weaken into the more troublesome Moderate category.

❏	❏	☑	❏
0	*1*	*2*	*3*
None	*Mild*	*Moderate*	*Severe*

IF A MAN does not take care of himself, then his score will worsen—drift upward—by about 25 to 100 points per year.

Score: 200 to 400 Moderate

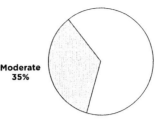

This is a more serious category. About 35 percent of the midlife men I see score in the Moderate range.

Men in this range know that something's up, that their milestone fortieth birthday has passed, and that nagging troubles are having effects.

They sense difficulties in a number of areas but are astonished at their own replies in the questionnaire. They will say, "You know, come to think of it, I am like that. I never really considered these things. And I'm not sure when or how it all happened."

This group tends to be the dumbfounded crowd, the ones wondering, "What is going on? I was able to get away with everything before—all those late nights, overeating, booze, overextending myself. But now, the body, mind, and soul seem to be protesting. Anyway, let me just push a little bit more, see what else I can get out of this machine. Hopefully it'll all go away on its own."

Fading Away Does Not Have to Be Part of Aging

The Moderate scoring group has a large share of "grin-and-bear-it" men. They may feel that many areas of their life are fading, and know they can't meet all their challenges. But they don't know why, or what to do. Playing macho, they don't admit—even to themselves—that they may need help and guidance.

They may have bought in to a doctor's common reassurance, "Don't worry, you're just getting old. What did you expect? Some things have to give out." With our current knowledge of male physiology—how a man's body works—this comforting reassurance is unacceptable.

It's actually saying, "Look, you're having a good life. But you have to accept what's coming. Less joy, less productivity, more pain of *all* kinds—physical and emotional—maybe bypass surgery, and your quota of prescription drugs. So what if you might need to pop pills to get it up? That's all part of the territory."

This group of men has to be reminded that there is such a thing as optimal functioning, as a prime of life, as full vitality and virility, and that they can regain it. These men still have positive relationships to help them get through their challenges and adopt new teachings from medical science. However, these men will be required to change—to think and behave in ways that they are not used to.

There is a wide range of scores in the Moderate category:

201 to 250 *low*-Moderate
251 to 350 *mid*-Moderate
351 to 400 *high*-Moderate

If you scored just above 200, you are at the entry level of the Moderate range. This is a *low*-Moderate score.

Your concerns are not as intense as the *high*-Moderate men, who score from 351 to 400.

The *high*-Moderate men are in trouble. For them, it means that *every* area important to men is affected:

- Changing body
- Sleep
- Sexuality
- Appearance
- Energy levels
- Medical background
- Habits and lifestyle
- Diet
- Changing personality
- Mind
- Stress levels
- Drive
- Self-esteem
- Happiness
- Relationships

These men, scoring close to 400, are beginning to go numb, beginning to distance themselves from their supports, and to shut down. They are beginning to get more comfort from being left alone, being hostile, or escaping into computers, TV, substance abuse, work, or spectator sports.

These are the men who have affairs with some new young thing to supercharge themselves. They think about cosmetic facial surgery, and buy red sports cars to be young again. With time, they give up positive pleasures for negative, unhealthy ones.

Depending on the Man's Willingness, He Will Respond to Advice

It is often rewarding to deal with this group of men, because the advice here leads to significant improvements, and most of these men *want* to be helped. They are pleased that their spouses accompany them to their appointments. They are grateful when they go through the questionnaire and begin the process of positive change.

Most men in the Moderate group are still willing to listen, and they haven't gone into hiding, into nasty, armored, protective shells—yet.

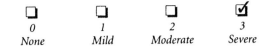

$$\begin{array}{cccc}
\square & \square & \square & \boxed{\checkmark} \\
0 & 1 & 2 & 3 \\
\textit{None} & \textit{Mild} & \textit{Moderate} & \textit{Severe}
\end{array}$$

Score: 401 to 500 Severe

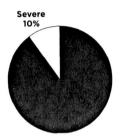

Severe
10%

This is the range of significant difficulty. Things are nasty. These men die many deaths even while living. About 10 percent of the midlife men I see score in this range.

These are the men who tend to be dragged in by an exhausted spouse, as if to say, "Please, for God's sake, help us."

These Men Perplex Their Health-Care Practitioners

Men in the Severe range confuse their health-care practitioners. Their X-rays are normal, and blood test panels may not show any significant problems. The electrocardiogram (EKG) might show some heart strain, but nothing to explain the grand list of complaints on the questionnaire.

If a doctor does ask about mood problems, the men reply that they are not especially sad or depressed. In fact, they are hostile. And doctors don't know what to do for that.

These men may get handed endless prescription drugs to chase individual symptoms. One drug for sleep, one for stress, one for cholesterol, one for blood pressure, one for aches and pains, one of the sons of Viagra for erections, and so on. They're told, "Take it easy, slow down. Maybe a specialist can help. Maybe you're just too stressed out and need a vacation."

This is the group of men who get (mis)diagnosed with full-blown clinical depression, who separate from their spouses, who find themselves in a rut at work, and who abuse themselves and others in so many ways.

And if they don't see a health-care practitioner, these are the men who suffer in ignorance at home and take down others with them, particularly their long-suffering loved ones. These men are asked by their spouses, "Don't you care about anything anymore?"

There Is Often an Outside Trigger

These men may have been coasting in the Moderate range for some time, even several years. But an outside event may have triggered their flare-up into the Severe range—they may have been physically injured, downsized from work, or suffered a financial loss or divorce.

These are the men:

- Whose stories end up in the movies, dealing with midlife crises, anger management, layoffs and downsizing, chilling divorces, weekend parenting, violence, addictions, alcoholism, and failure.
- Who overuse substances to self-medicate, to escape.
- Who act out, stay angry, scream a lot, and mean it when they tell everyone to go to hell.
- Who will make sure that men continue to die seven to ten years earlier than women.

These men need devoted help, and to follow the advice in this book closely. It can be done, but it requires a thick-skinned team. And it starts with the individual man, who must be motivated to make the necessary changes to help himself.

UNDERSTAND THE NUANCES IN THIS QUESTIONNAIRE AND ITS SCORING

Questionnaires such as this one are to be used for self-assessment, to bring points forward for discussion, to help all concerned, and to alert clients and their loved ones to issues that need to be managed. These scores serve as a guide.

Men Can Be Disappointed by Their Scores for Various Reasons

Some men are upset that they got a *good*, low score, only in the Mild range. They were looking for an explanation, perhaps also something to blame their circumstances on. "See dear, that's what's going on. I got this male menopause thing. And you're the one causing it."

Some men who score in the Severe range get very agitated, even tearful. They take home the message that life is over. Some even make their wills, and it may take a couple of encounters for us to debrief them.

One of the toughest groups to deal with is the men who don't care, even after they have scored in the Severe range. These men seem to be irreversibly hostile, and resent even being in our offices. They disregard the assessment and advice entirely, can't be bothered, and think that they are wasting their time. "So what, Dr. Q? Tell me something I didn't already know."

These are the men who swear at the staff as they stomp out of the clinic.

There Can Be Unanticipated Nuances to the Questions

Some men get hung up on the language. For example, consider the question "Are you getting overweight, adding a new layer of fat around your waist?" Some men ask, "Well, how do I know if it's a new or old layer of fat?"

Some questions reveal a lot about the men by accident. Consider the questions "Is your *partner* less sexually satisfied?" or "Are the number or intensity of your *partner's* orgasms less? Men say, "How should I know? I don't *ask*. You want me to do quality control?"

Obviously, these men need to communicate more openly with their partners, which I encourage.

FOLLOW *ALL* THE CHAPTERS, BUT PAY SPECIAL ATTENTION TO THE CORE RECOMMENDATIONS BASED ON YOUR SCORE

Score: 0 to 50 None

Men in this category who have specific issues to work through—such as obesity, diabetes, or sex issues—should concentrate on those specific chapters regardless of what their scores are.

Even if you scored in the good, None category, continue to take the questionnaire annually. Also, if there are subsections, such as sleep or sexuality, for which you did have significant scores, follow the recommendations in the related chapters to improve your scores in those areas.

Score: 51 to 200 Mild

Pay special attention to the core recommendations in the following chapters:

- Chapter 2   Sleep
- Chapter 3   Sex
- Chapter 4   Exercise
- Chapter 6   Diet
- Chapter 13 Stress Levels

Score: 201 to 400 Moderate

Pay special attention to the core recommendations in the following chapters:

- Chapter 2   Sleep
- Chapter 3   Sex
- Chapter 4   Exercise
- Chapter 6   Diet

- Chapter 7   Heart Trouble
- Chapter 8   Obesity
- Chapter 10 Supplements
- Chapter 13 Stress Levels
- Chapter 16 Relationships

Score: 401 to 500 Severe
Severe-end men will need to closely follow the advice in all these chapters:

- Chapter 2   Sleep
- Chapter 3   Sex
- Chapter 4   Exercise
- Chapter 6   Diet
- Chapter 7   Heart Trouble
- Chapter 8   Obesity
- Chapter 9   Diabetes
- Chapter 10 Supplements
- Chapter 11 Genital and Urinary Systems
- Chapter 13 Stress Levels
- Chapter 14 Therapeutic Self-Massage
- Chapter 15 Workplace
- Chapter 16 Relationships
- Chapter 17 Spirituality and Health

TAKE THE FULL T-QUESTIONNAIRE ONCE A YEAR TO MONITOR CHANGES AND YOUR DRIFTING SCORE

Scores change.

From one year to the next, scores can drift upward—worsen—from 25 to 100 points. That can easily change your ranking—from Mild to Moderate, or Moderate to Severe. So it's important to do a "yearly tune-up" as part of a regular maintenance program, to track these changes.

Then you can implement more of the recommendations in this book as they are needed.

Bibliography

BOOKS

Allen, Tim. *I'm Not Really Here.* New York: Warner Books, 1997.

Alman, Brian, Ph.D., and Peter Lambrou. *Self-Hypnosis: A Complete Manual for Health and Self-Change.* San Diego: International Health Publications, 1983.

Bain, Jerald, M.D., ed. *Mechanisms in Andropause.* Concord, Ontario: Mechanisms in Medicine Inc., 2003.

Benson, Herbert, M.D. *Timeless Healing: The Power and Biology of Belief.* New York: Scribner, 1997.

Bowskill, Derek, and Anthea Linacre. *The 'Male' Menopause.* London: Frederick Muller Limited, 1976.

Brand-Miller, Jennie, Ph.D., and Wolever, Thomas, Ph.D., et al. *The New Glucose Revolution: The Authoritative Guide to the Glycemic Index—the Dietary Solution for Lifelong Health.* New York: Marlowe & Company, 2002.

Buford, Bob. *Halftime: Changing Your Game Plan from Success to Significance.* Grand Rapids, MI: Zondervan Publishing House, 1994.

Burton Nelson, Mariah. *The Stronger Women Get, the More Men Love Football: Sexism and the American Culture of Sports.* New York: Avon Books, 1994.

Byron, Christopher. *Testosterone, Inc: Tales of CEOs Gone Wild.* Hoboken, NJ: Wiley, 2004.

Carruthers, Malcolm, M.D. *Androgen Deficiency in the Adult Male: Causes, Diagnosis, and Treatment.* London, UK: Taylor & Francis Group, 2004.

———. *Maximising Manhood: Beating the Male Menopause.* London, UK: Harper-Collins Publishers, 1996.

———. *The Testosterone Revolution: Rediscover Your Energy and Overcome the Symptoms of Male Menopause.* London, UK: Thorsons Publishing, 2001.

Cetel, Nancy, M.D. *Double Menopause: What To Do When Both of You and Your Mate Go Through Hormonal Changes Together.* Hoboken, NJ: Wiley, 2002.

Courter, Gay, and Pat Gaudette. *How to Survive Your Husband's Midlife Crisis.* New York: The Berkley Publishing Group, 2003.

Crowley, Chris, and Henry S. Lodge, M.D. *Younger Next Year: A Guide to Living Like 50 Until You're 80 and Beyond.* New York: Workman Publishing, 2004.

Currie, Shawn, Ph.D., and Keith Wilson, Ph.D. *Sleep-Ease: Quick Tips to Get a Good Night's Rest.* Far Hills, NJ: New Horizon Press, 2002.

Dabbs, James M., Ph.D., and Mary G. Dabbs. *Heroes, Rogues, and Lovers: Testosterone and Behavior.* New York: McGraw-Hill, 2000.

Dane, Lance, ed. *The Complete Illustrated Kama Sutra.* Rochester, VT: Inner Traditions, 2003.

Davidson, Jeff. *The Complete Idiot's Guide to Managing Stress.* Indianapolis, IN: Alpha Books, 1999.

de Kruif, Paul. *The Male Hormone.* New York: Harcourt, Brace, & Company, 1945.

Diamond, Jed, Ph.D. *Male Menopause.* Naperville, IL: Sourcebooks, Inc., 1998.

———. *Surviving Male Menopause: A Guide for Women and Men.* Naperville, IL: Sourcebooks, Inc., 2000.

———. *The Irritable Male Syndrome.* Emmaus, PA.: Rodale, 2004.

Dossey, Larry, M.D. *Healing Words: The Power of Prayer and the Practice of Medicine.* San Francisco: HarperSanFrancisco, 1994.

———. *Reinventing Medicine: Beyond Mind-Body to a New Era of Healing.* San Francisco: HarperSanFrancisco, 1999.

Elkin, Allen, Ph.D., *Stress Management for Dummies.* New York: Wiley Publishing, Inc., 1999.

Fisch, Harry, M.D., and Stephen Braun. *The Male Biological Clock: The Startling News About Aging, Sexuality, and Fertility in Men.* New York: Free Press, 2005.

Gallop, Rick. *The G.I. Diet: The Easy, Healthy Way to Permanent Weight Loss.* Toronto: Random House Canada, 2002.

Giampapa, Vincent, M.D., and Ronald Pero, Ph.D., et al. *The Anti-Aging Solution: 5 Simple Steps to Looking and Feeling Young.* Hoboken, NJ: Wiley, 2004.

Gurian, Michael. *What Could He Be Thinking? How a Man's Mind Really Works.* New York: St. Martin's Press, 2003.

Goldman, Robert, M.D., and Ronald Klatz, M.D. *The New Anti-Aging Revolution: Stopping the Clock for a Younger, Sexier, Happier YOU!* North Bergen, NJ: Basic Health Publications, 2003.

Gray, Henry. *Gray's Anatomy*, 15th Revised Edition. New York: Gramercy, 1988.

Hallberg, Edmond C. *The Gray Itch: The Male Metapause Syndrome.* New York: Stein and Day Publishers, 1978.

Harbin, Thomas J., Ph.D. *Beyond Anger: A Guide for Men.* New York: Marlowe & Company, 2000.

Hill, Aubrey M., M.D. *Viropause/Andropause, The Male Menopause: Emotional and Physical Changes Mid-life Men Experience.* Far Hills, NJ: New Horizon Press, 1993.

Hister, Art, M.D. *Dr. Art Hister's Guide to Living A Long & Healthy Life.* Vancouver: Greystone Books, 2003.

———. *Midlife Man: A not-so-threatening guide to health and sex for man at his peak.* Vancouver: Greystone Books, 1998.

Hunter, Marlene, M.D. *Psych Yourself In! Hypnosis & Health.* Vancouver: SeaWalk Press Ltd., 1987.

Jones, Marcia, Ph.D., and Theresa Eichenwald, M.D. *Menopause for Dummies.* New York: Wiley Publishing, Inc., 2003.

Kagan, Leslee, and Bruce Kessel, M.D., et al. *Mind Over Menopause: The Complete Mind/Body Approach to Coping with Menopause.* New York: Free Press, 2004.

Kaufman, Francine, M.D. *Diabesity: the Obesity-Diabetes Epidemic That Threatens America—And What We Must Do to Stop It.* New York: Bantam, 2005.

Khan, S. N., *Psychology of the Hero Soul: Promoting Heroes in the Workplace & Everyday Life.* Toronto: Diamond Mind Publishing, 2004.

Kita, Joe, et al. *Guy Q: 1,305 Totally Essential Secrets You Either Know, or You Don't.* Emmaus, PA: Rodale, 2003.

Koenig, Harold G., M.D. *The Healing Power of Faith.* New York: Touchstone Books, 2001.

Koenig, Harold G., M.D., and Michael E. McCullough, Ph.D., et al. *Handbook of Religion and Health.* Oxford, UK: Oxford University Press, 2000.

Love, Susan, M.D., and Karen Lindsey. *Dr. Susan Love's Menopause & Hormone Book.* New York: Three Rivers Press, 2003.

Marsh, F. Chapin. *The Faith Factor.* Mosheim, TN: Black Forest Press, 2004.

Maté, Gabor, M.D. *When the Body Says No: The Cost of Hidden Stress.* Toronto: Vintage Canada, 2004.

Meryn, Siegfried, M.D., and Markus Metka, M.D., et al. *Men's Health & the Hormone Revolution.* Vienna, Austria: NDE Publishing, 2000.

Nedd, Kenford, M.D., *Power Over Stress: 35 Quick Prescriptions for Mastering the Stress in Your Life.* Toronto: QP Press, 2004.

Nieschlag, Eberhard, M.D., and H.M. Behre, M.D., eds. *Testosterone: Action, Deficiency, Substitution.* Cambridge, UK: Cambridge University Press, 2004.

O'Connor, Richard, Ph.D., *Undoing Perpetual Stress: The Missing Connection Between Depression, Anxiety, and 21st Century Illness.* New York: The Berkley Publishing Group, 2005.

Porter, Roy, Ph.D., *The Greatest Benefit to Mankind: A Medical History of Humanity.* New York: W.W. Norton & Company, 1999.

Pressman, Alan, Ph.D., and Sheila Buff. *The Complete Idiot's Guide to Vitamins and Minerals.* Indianapolis, IN: Alpha Books, 2000.

Rabin, Bruce. *Stress, Immune Function, and Health: The Connection.* Hoboken, NJ: John Wiley & Sons, 1999.

Real, Terrence. *I Don't Want to Talk About It: Overcoming the Secret Legacy of Male Depression.* New York: Scribner, 1997.

Rippe, James, M.D. *Heart Disease for Dummies.* New York: Wiley Publishing, Inc., 2004

Scardino, Peter T., M.D., and Judith Kelman. *Dr. Peter Scardino's Prostate Book: The Complete Guide to Overcoming Prostate Cancer, Prostatitis, and BPH.* New York: Avery Publishing Group, Inc., 2005.

Schuler, Lou, and Jeff Volek, Ph.D., et al. *The Testosterone Advantage Plan: Lose Weight, Gain Muscle, Boost Energy.* Emmaus, PA: Rodale, 2002.

Schwarzbein, Diana, M.D., and Marilyn Brown. *The Schwarzbein Principle II: A Regeneration Process to Prevent and Reverse Accelerated Aging.* Deerfield Beach, FL: Health Communications, Inc., 2002.

Segal, Sheldon, Ph.D., and Luigi Mastroianni Jr., M.D. *Hormone Use in Menopause and Male Andropause: A Choice for Women and Men.* Oxford, UK: Oxford University Press, 2003.

Senay, Emily, M.D., and Rob Walters. *From Boys to Men: A Woman's Guide to the Health of Husbands, Partners, Sons, Fathers, and Brothers.* New York: Scribner, 2004.

Sheehy, Gail. *The Silent Passage: Revised and Updated Edition.* New York: Pocket Books, 1998.

———. *Understanding Men's Passages: Discovering the New Map of Men's Lives.* New York: Ballantine Books, 1999.

Shippen, Eugene, M.D., and William Fryer. *The Testosterone Syndrome: The Critical Factor for Energy, Love, & Sexuality—Reversing the Male Menopause.* New York: M. Evans and Company, Inc., 1998.

Seigel, Bernie, M.D. *Love, Medicine, and Miracles.* New York: HarperCollins, 1990.

Simon, Harvey B., M.D. *The Harvard Medical School Guide to Men's Health.* New York: Free Press, 2004.

Somers, Suzanne. *The Sexy Years.* New York: Crown Publishers, 2004.

Tafler, David. *50+ Survival Guide: Winning Strategies for Wealth, Health, and Lifestyle.* Toronto: ITP Nelson, 1998.

Tan, Robert, M.D. *The Andropause Mystery: Unraveling Truths About the Male Menopause.* Houston: Amred Consulting, 2001.

Wolfe, Tom. *A Man in Full.* New York: Bantam Books, 2001.

———. *The Bonfire of the Vanities.* New York: Bantam Books, 1990.

Zimmerman, Marcia. *Eat Your Colors: Maximize Your Health by Eating the Right Foods For Your Body Type.* New York: Owl Books, 2001.

ARTICLES

Blumentals, W., M.D. and A. Gomez-Caminero, Ph.D., et al. "Is Erectile Dysfunction Predictive of Peripheral Vascular Disease?" *The Aging Male* 6:217–221, 2003.

Casey, Richard, M.D., ed. *Journal of Sexual & Reproductive Medicine,* Autumn 2001.

Cauli, O., Ph.D., and M. Morelli, Ph.D. "Caffeine and the Dopaminergic System." *Behavioral Pharmacology* 17:2, May 1992.

Diczfalusy, E., M.D. "The Aging Male and Developed Countries in the 21st Century." *The Aging Male* 5:139–146, 2002.

Dowd, Maureen. "Men Just Want Mommy." *New York Times* (Op-Ed), January 13, 2005.

Dunajska, K., M.D., and A. Milewicz, M.D. "Evaluation of Sex Hormone Levels and Some Metabolic Factors in Men with Coronary Atherosclerosis." *The Aging Male,* 7:197–204, 2004.

Fredholm, B. B., Ph.D. "Adenosine, Adenosine Receptors, and the Actions of Caffeine." *Pharmacological Toxicology* 76:2, February 1995.

Gooren, L. J. G., M.D. "Visceral Obesity, Androgens and the Risks of Cardiovascular Disease and Diabetes Mellitus." *The Aging Male* 4:30–38, 2001.

Heinemann, L. A. J., M.D., and F. Saad, M.D., et al. "Can Results of the Aging Males' Symptoms (AMS) Scale Predict Those of Screening Scales for Androgen Deficiency?" *The Aging Male* 7:211–18, 2004.

Hodges, F. M., Ph.D. "The Penalties of Passion and Desire: Love and the Aging Male in Early 20th-Century Film." *The Aging Male* 6:222–29, 2003.

Karolkiewicz, J., Ph.D., and L. Szczesniak, Ph.D., et al. "Oxidative stress and Antioxidant Defense System in Healthy, Elderly Men: Relationship to Physical Activity." *The Aging Male* 6:100–105, 2003.

Kaufman, J. M., M.D. and G. T'Sjoen, Ph.D. "The Effects of Testosterone Deficiency on Male Sexual Function." *The Aging Male* 5:242–47, 2002.

Lister, Sam. "Careful, Lads, That Laptop Might Burn Your Genes." *Times Online* (UK), December 9, 2004. www.timesonline.co.uk/article/0,,2-1395183,00.html.

Marandola, P., M.D. and S. Musitelli, M.D., et al. "Love and Sexuality in Aging." *The Aging Male* 5:103–13, 2002.

Nehlig, A., Ph.D., and J. L. Daval, Ph.D. "Caffeine and the Central Nervous System: Mechanisms of Action, Biochemical, Metabolic and Psychostimulant Effects." *Brain Research Review* 17:2, May 1992.

Notzon, F. C., M.D., and Y. M. Komarov, M.D., et al. "Causes of Declining Life Expectancy in Russia." *Journal of the American Medical Association* (*JAMA*) 279:10, March 1998.

Ostrowska, B., Ph.D., and K. Rozek-Mroz, Ph.D., et al. "Body Posture in Elderly, Physically Active Males." *The Aging Male,* 6:222-229, 2003.

Qaadri, Shafiq, M.D. "When Men Go through the Change." *Globe and Mail,* January 22, 2002.

———. "Bred in the Bone." *Globe and Mail,* November 26, 2002.

———. "Why We Can't Sleep It All Off." *Globe and Mail,* February 5, 2002.

———. "All about Andropause." *Medical Post,* October 8, 2002.

———. "Andropause: A Man's Menopause." *Canadian Journal of Diagnosis,* May 2002.

Sheynkin, Yefim, M.D., and Michael Jung, M.D. "Increase in Scrotal Temperature in Laptop Computer Users." *Human Reproduction.* 20:2, December 2004.

Swan, S. H., Ph.D., and E. P. Elkin. Ph.D. "The Question of Declining Sperm Density Revisited: An Analysis of 101 Studies Published 1934–1996." *Environmental Health Perspectives* 108:10, October 2000.

———., et al. "Have Sperm Densities Declined? A Reanalysis of Global Trend Data." *Environmental Health Perspectives* 105:11, November 1997.

Svenningsson, Per, Ph.D., and George G. Nomikos, Ph.D., et al. "The Stimulatory Action and the Development of Tolerance to Caffeine Is Associated with Alterations in Gene Expression in Specific Brain Regions." *Journal of Neuroscience* 19:10, May 15, 1999.

WEB SITES

American Academy of Anti-Aging Medicine: www.worldhealth.net

American Diabetes Association: www.diabetes.org

American Heart Association: www.americanheart.org

American Music Therapy Association: www.musictherapy.org

American Stroke Association: www.strokeassociation.org

Centre University Andropause 101: http://centeru.com/andropause.html

Duke University Centre for Spirituality, Theology, and Health: www.dukespiritualityandhealth.org

The Environmental Working Group: The Power of Information: www.ewg.org
Home of the Glycemic Index: www.glycemicindex.com
Heart and Stroke Foundation of Canada: www.heartandstroke.ca
International Society for the Study of the Aging Male: www.issam.ch
The John D. and Catherine T. MacArthur Foundation Research Network on Successful Midlife Development (MIDMAC): http://midmac.med.harvard.edu
Life Extension Foundation: www.lef.org
Men's Health Magazine: menshealth.com
U.S. Food and Drug Administration: Department of Health and Human Services: www.fda.gov

Index

abdominal fat, 98, 100, 111
adrenaline, 158
age forty, 88–89, 204
air bicycle, 39
alcohol, 69, 215
Allen, Woody, 26
amino acids, 100
anger, 162
angina, 31
antibiotics, 146
apologizing, 214–15
appearance, 34, 241
arguments, 210–11, 214–15
aromatase enzyme, 76
ascending infection, 142
aspirin (ASA), 121–22

baby boomers, ix, x, 270
benzophenone, 71
bladder, 144
blood pressure, 64, 89–91
body image, 233–35, 241
bones, 101, 126–27
brain-testes connection, xii
breakfast, 79
breast cancer, 71
breathing, 161

caffeine, 67–69
calcium, 101, 126–27
cancer, 70–71, 120
carbohydrates, 118
cardiovascular disease, 31–32, 64, 81–94
celery, 76
chancroid, 142
cheating, 202, 207

chemicals, 71
chin tuck, 161–62
chlamydia, 138, 141, 146–47
cholesterol, 89–90, 92, 94, 100
Clinton, Bill, 78
communication, 211–12
condoms, 146
cortisol, 158–59
cytochrome p450 enzyme system, 77

dental care, 83
diabetes, 105–18
diet, 55–80, 247–48
doctors, 231
Dossey, Larry, 219
drive, 172–75, 254–55

EKG (electrocardiogram), 91
energy, 242
epididymis, 144
erectile dysfunction (ED), 29–32, 88
estrogen, 70–71, 76, 99–102, 129
exercise, 33–45

faith, 217–25
family, 195–96
fast-food, 78
fasting glucose, 114
fasting insulin, 116
fasting rituals, 224
fat, 98, 100–1
fatty acids, 100
fertility, 147
fever, 174
fiber, 75
fidgeting, 45

fish, 70–73
fish oils, 129–31
flex gluteals, 43
folic acid supplements, 123
food, 55–80, 247–48
food pyramid, 59–60
foreplay, 25–26
fruits, 70–75

genital human papilloma virus, 141–42
genital system, 136–48
glucosuria, 116–17
glycemic index, 118
glycogen, 101
gonorrhea, 142, 147
grapefruit, 76
green tea, 68
gum disease, 83
gynecomastia, 102

habits, 52–53, 245–46
happiness, 261–62
Hawaii relaxation script, 164
heart disease, 31–32, 64, 81–94
heat production, 113
hemoglobin A1c, 92, 114–15
herbal supplements, 135
herpes, 138–39, 141
high blood pressure, 64, 89–91
high-sensitivity C-reactive protein
    (hsC-RP), 93
homocysteine, 93, 123
hormone production system, xi
hormones, 70, 158
hypertension, 64, 89–91

indole-3-carbinol (I3C), 133–35
infertility, 111, 139, 175
infidelity, 202, 207
insulin, 109–12, 116, 131
jealousy, 207–9

jobs, 183–96
jumping squat, 39

kegel exercises, 43
kidneys, 144

laptop computers, 176–77
leptins, 102–3
lifestyle, 52–53, 245–46
liver, 76

massage, 179–82
masturbation, 26–27, 146
meat, 70–72

medical background, 49–51, 243–44
melengestrol, 70
mental state, 153–54, 251
Metformin, 111
microalbuminuria, 117
microbial infections, 137–48
middle-age spread, 98–99, 111
midlife crisis, 204
milk, 78
minerals, 101, 119–35
multivitamin, 122–24, 132
muscle-tension sweep, 164–68

nettle root extract, 133–35
nitrates, 31
nutritional guidelines, 59–60

obesity, 77, 91, 95–104
oils, 78
omega-3&6, 129–31
oral sex, 27, 139
orgasm, 22–24
osteoporosis, 126–27
overweight, 77, 91, 95–104
oxygen, 203–4
oxyphenone, 71
oysters, 76

pelvic cardio exercise, 38–40
pelvic circle, 40
pelvic resistance exercise, 40–44
pelvic thrust, 39–42
perineum, 179–81
peripheral artery disease, 110
personality changes, 151–52, 249–50
pheromones, 23
phthalate, 72
phytoestrogens, 77
polycystic ovarian syndrome, 110–11
portion sizes, 59–61
postprandial glucose spikes, 115
potbelly, 111
poultry, 72
prayer, 221
prehypertension, 90
progesterone, 70
prostate, 144–45
proteins, 100
puberty, xi
pudendal nerve, 178

questionnaire, 3–4, 229–76
    scoring, 263–76

relationships, 197–216, 258–60
religion, 217–25

salt, 63–65
seafood, 70–73
selenium, 128
self-esteem, 168–69, 183–96, 256–57
self-massage, 179–82
sex, 18–32, 237–40
sexual hygiene, 146–47
sexually transmitted disease (STD), 138–48
SHBG (sex-hormone binding globulin),
    110
shopping therapy, 170
shoulder roll, 162
sitting ergonomics, 177–79
sleep, 8–17, 104, 236–37
smoking, 120
snacks, 75
soy, 77
sperm count, xii, 24, 174–75
spices, 77
spirituality, 217–25
sports, 195
starches, 61–63
stress, 155–70, 252–53
stroke, 64
subclinical infections, 139
sugar, 61–63, 105, 109, 118
supplements, 119–35
syndrome X, 111–17

tea, 68
temperature of testes, 174–77
thermogenesis, 113

thigh workout, 42
trenbolone, 70
triglycerides, 92, 117

urethra, 144
urinary system, 136–48
urine, 116–17, 147, 182
urine test, 148
vegetables, 70–75

Viagra, 31, 89
visualization techniques, 163–69
vitamins, 119–35
    vitamin B, 132–33
    vitamin C, 127–28
    vitamin D, 128–29
    vitamin E, 131–32

waist measurement, 91, 98
water, 65–67, 147
weight, 77, 91, 95–104
weight chart, 96–97
weight loss, 103–4
women, ix, 206
    infertility, 111, 139
workplace, 183–96

xenoestrogens, 77

zeranol, 70
zinc, 76, 125